Hey, I Can Make It!
Plant Based.

The DAREBEE Cookbook

2021

N. Rey | darebee.com

First Printing, 2021.
ISBN 13: 978-1-84481-160-1
ISBN 10: 1-84481-160-3

Published by New Line Books, London

Warning and Disclaimer
Although every precaution has been taken to verify the accuracy of the information contained herein, the author and publisher assume no responsibility for any errors or omissions. No liability is assumed for damage or injury that may result from the use of information contained within.

Author Bio

Neila Rey is the founder of Darebee, a global fitness resource. She is committed to democratizing fitness by removing the barriers to it and increasing accessibility. Every workout published in her books utilizes the latest in exercise science and has undergone thorough field testing and refinement through Darebee volunteers. When she's not busy running Darebee she is focused on finding fresh ways to make exercise easier and more enjoyable.

In keeping with the philosophy of Darebee this cookbook is also the result of extensive field trials. Its basic principle is accessibility and ease of use. Its focus is on fitness and nutrition as well as health and tasty cooking.

Index

Introduction

Welcome to the Darebee cookbook! All the recipes in this book are easy and quick to make and require next to no cooking skills and minimal kitchen equipment. They are also all made in a healthy way with a focus on fitness and maximum nutrition for overall well-being.

This collection consists of everyday dishes, something you would make regularly for breakfast, lunch and dinner. It will help you decide what to make every single day and make meal planning easy. The same ingredients come up again and again so food shopping should also become less of a hustle.

Feel free to modify the recipes to better suit your taste, add extra spices and garnish the way you like. You can also swap ingredients based on what you have in your fridge and pantry. To help you, we've added a section at the back of this book where you can record your notes and shortcuts to your favorite recipes.

When choosing recipes for this book we wanted you to actually feel you can make them but at the same time make them interesting and exciting to look at. We also spent time putting together combinations of foods that a) are not going to break the bank b) will give you the best nutrition when combined.

All of the recipes in this book are healthy and are all designed to help you reach and maintain your fitness goals.

How to use this book

Each recipe gives you three portion sizes: small, medium and large.

Pick a small portion size, if:

- You are trying to reduce your body fat percentage and your daily caloric intake in general;
- You are not used to eating big meals or you eat micro meals throughout the day;
- You had a large meal earlier in the day and don't feel like eating a lot;
- You are having other dishes like salads, bread and/or dessert with your meal.

A medium portion size is your regular plate for every day. Choose it, if:

- You are exercising regularly and you are just trying to streamline or maintain your body fat percentage;
- You are trying to build muscle tone while also trying to drop body fat;
- You are eating three times a day and this is one of your meals.

A large portion size is for you, if:

- You are trying to gain weight and put on muscle. You don't want to lose body fat;
- You eat one or two meals a day.

The recipes for each portion size were not just increased based on quantity but with a focus on extra protein and the ingredients containing it. We designed the portion system also based on how you cook and the ingredients you will be using so you don't end up with half an apple in the fridge or are forced to open an extra can of beans.

When cooking for two or more people simply multiply the portions you are making by the number of people you are cooking for. Remember, though, the recipes and the quantities given in this book are all guidelines only. You are the master of your kitchen, you make the rules. This book was designed to make your life easier, give you ideas and help you feel more in control.

Toppings

At the end of each recipe you will find a step prompting you to top and garnish every dish you make. Usually we will recommend fresh herbs, spices, nuts and seeds but if you don't have any on hand or you just aren't a fan of a particular topping, just skip it or change it. The reason we all should try to make our dishes look Instagram-worthy is because our brains are hardwired to respond to colourful and interesting food.

When we see food that looks good, we begin to secrete digestive juices in anticipation. We can then better absorb what we eat and get maximum nutrition from the same food when it's presented in a more appetising manner. How we feel about what we eat is just as important as what we eat. Food should make us feel happy and satisfied every time.

Salt

All recipes in this book are given without any salt. That's because the saltiness of food is a very personal matter. Some people prefer things to be very salty and others like it less. With so many people reducing their salt intake the margin for error in any given recipe is incredibly high. So, season for taste. Either add salt as you go while making recipes from this book or add it as a final touch. Alternatively serve your dishes with a bottle of soy sauce on the side. A dash of soy sauce will liven up any rice dish or soup in an instant.

Maple Syrup & Molasses

We are using molasses and maple syrup as sweeteners in this book but you are free to replace them with one of your choice.

The reason we use blackstrap molasses is because as far as sweeteners go it's one of the best ones in terms of its nutritional value. Unlike regular sugar, blackstrap molasses is rich in iron, selenium, and copper, and even has some calcium in it. And it's cheap! So it's great value for money, too. Because you need very little each time one jar will go a long way. It works beautifully with all types of tomato, fresh tomatoes or tomato paste balancing out that sourness.

Maple syrup is our second sweetener of choice because of its subtle taste. You can use any other syrup instead of it like date, coconut or agave syrup. You can even use plain sugar - simply half the amount required for the recipe.

Tomato Paste vs Tomato Sauce vs Fresh Tomatoes

Sometimes a recipe calls for a little bit of umami taste and that's where tomatoes come in. It's not always possible or practical to use a fresh one so you should always have tomato paste in your pantry, ready to go on short notice. The reason we recommend you buy tomato paste is because it is essentially a concentrate sold in small quantities. It does go a long way.

Tomato sauces on the other hand are recommended for recipes where you need a large quantity of tomatoes. Once a jar is opened, you should either use up half of it or all of it. When you buy tomato sauce it often comes in different flavors like basil or olive or mushrooms which is an excellent shortcut for better tasting food.

And fresh tomatoes are best saved for fresh salads or for when you want to add extra chunkiness to your dishes. Canned chopped tomatoes will work here, too.

Beans

Plant based recipes often include lots of different beans because of their excellent nutritional value and good rep when it comes to health and longevity. All beans are nutritional powerhouses. They are high in protein, fiber and essential minerals. They are filling, comforting and tasty even on their own. The only drawback when it comes to beans is the need to soak them before cooking. It's an important step and it should not be skipped but yes, it's a hustle and it does mean that you have to plan your meals in advance. There are a couple of shortcuts for this.

Use canned beans. Bonus - they are already cooked and you can make meals with them in minutes. The drawback, it's more expensive in the long run and the texture of the beans is not quite the same.

Cook in bulk. This is especially useful if you are cooking for two or more people regularly. Soak and then cook a whole pack of beans in advance and keep them in a tupperware in the fridge. Then use them up throughout the week. Bulk cooking also works for grains and legumes. You can cook rice, lentils and quinoa and even sweet potatoes in large quantities in advance this way.

If you cook beans often a pressure cooker is a worthwhile investment. It's a set and forget solution. You can soak beans inside, drain and rinse them the next day then add fresh water and have them ready in 10-15 minutes. Pressure cookers are brilliant for all things beans. They will also cook rice, though, the best type of rice to cook in one is brown long grain Basmati rice. It comes out perfect every time.

Note: you can cook beans in pressure cookers without soaking but there are split opinions on that one. If you can, always soak beans before cooking.

Plant Based Dairy

All recipes in this cookbook use plant based dairy: milk, cream, cheese and yogurt. We often use cashew milk, cashew or soy cream and yogurt and cheese made from nuts in the DAREBEE kitchen. The type of dairy you use is up to you. Use what you have on hand or use what you simply prefer. We prefer cashew milk and cream because of its mild taste and turn to soy when we want creamier and richer texture.

Cooking Without Oil

You will notice that we saute, boil and roast everything in this cookbook and we rarely use oil, if at all. We use water. Cooking this way drastically reduces the overall Caloric value of all of the dishes and makes the clean up afterwards a breeze. Cooking with oil is mostly a habit for most of us but once you try cooking without it, food cooked with oil begins to taste heavy and not that tasty. If you want to cook with oil, though, that's ok too! Sometimes it is necessary to bring out certain flavours in food or create that golden crusty look.

Good quality oils, olive or avocado oils, should be reserved for salads or added to dishes after you are done cooking them to preserve all of their nutrients.

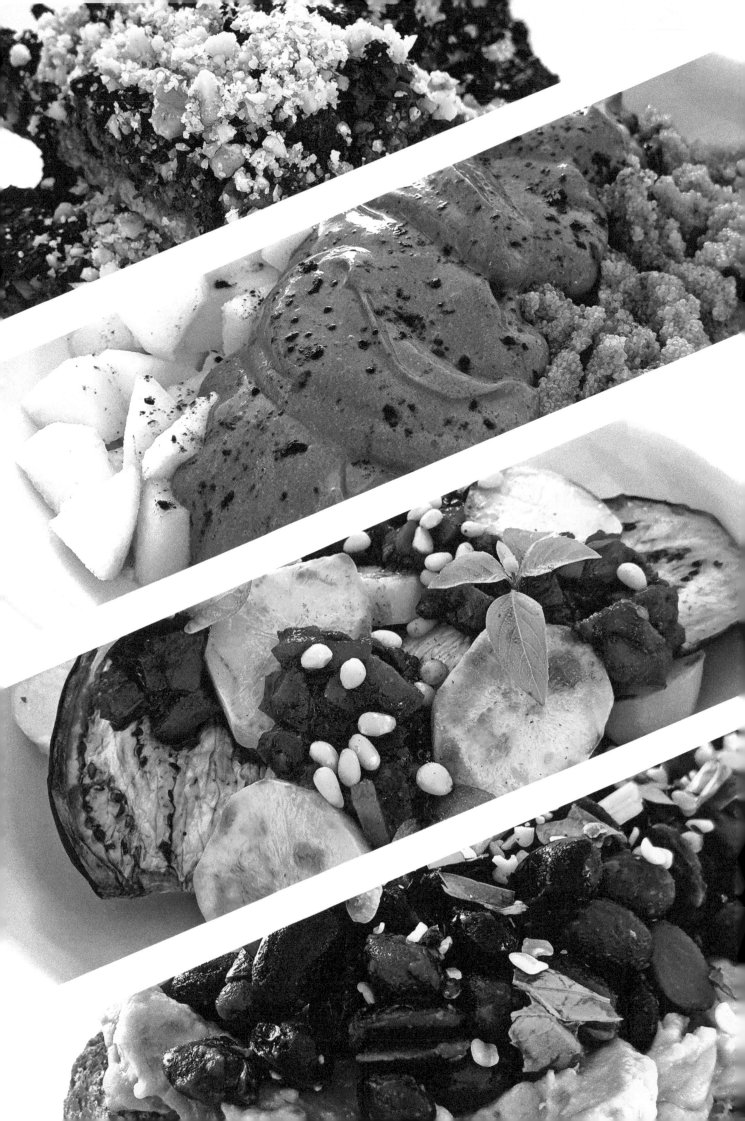

"Taste is a sensation enjoyed by the entire body and mind."

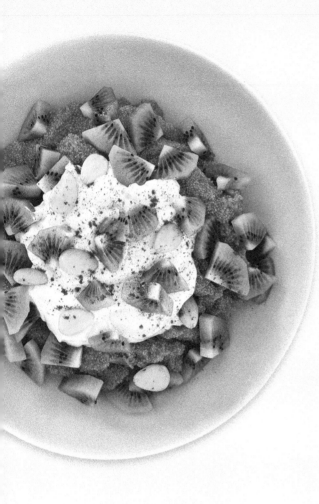

Amaranth With Yogurt & Kiwifruit

Visual Recipe
by DAREBEE
© darebee.com

	SMALL	MEDIUM	LARGE
amaranth	⅓ cup ~ 70g	½ cup ~ 100g	1 cup ~ 200g
plain yogurt	4oz ~ 120ml	6oz ~ 180ml	8oz ~ 240ml
kiwifruit	1	2	2

LEVEL UP! Add almonds and nutmeg.

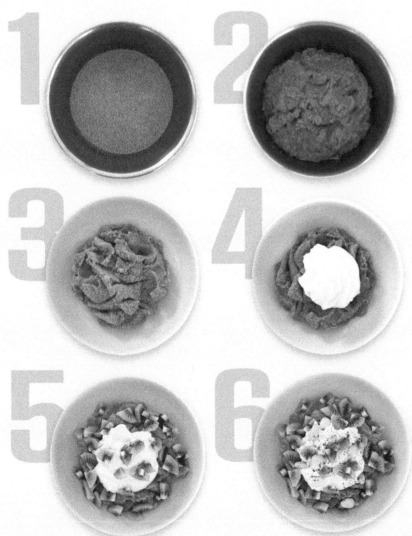

INSTRUCTIONS

1. Add amaranth to a cooking pot. Cover amaranth with double the amount of water and season for taste.

2. Bring water to a boil then lower heat to low. Cover the pot with a lid and simmer until it has completely absorbed the water ~ 15 minutes. The amaranth is cooked when it's no longer crunchy.

3. Transfer cooked amaranth to a plate.

4. Add yogurt.

5. Add peeled and sliced kiwifruit.

6. Top with almonds and sprinkle with nutmeg.

BREAKFAST

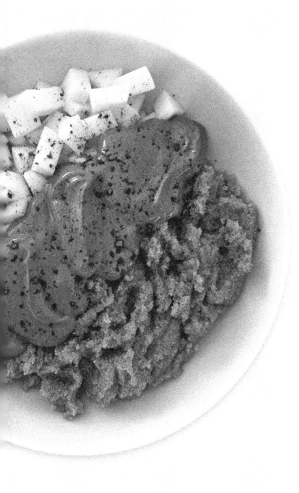

Amaranth With Yogurt & Pear

Visual Recipe
by DAREBEE
© darebee.com

	SMALL	MEDIUM	LARGE
amaranth	⅓ cup ~ 70g	½ cup ~ 100g	1 cup ~ 200g
plain yogurt	4oz ~ 120ml	6oz ~ 180ml	8oz ~ 240ml
pear	1	2	2
cocoa	½ tbsp	1 tbsp	2 tbsp

LEVEL UP! Use carob flour instead of cocoa powder.

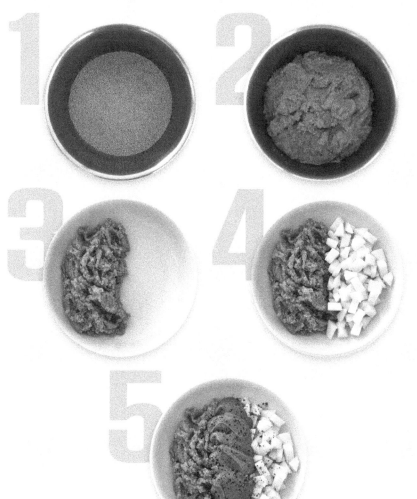

INSTRUCTIONS

1. Add amaranth to a cooking pot. Cover amaranth with double the amount of water and season for taste.

2. Bring water to a boil then lower heat to low. Cover the pot with a lid and simmer until it has completely absorbed the water ~ 15 minutes. The amaranth is cooked when it's no longer crunchy.

3. Transfer cooked amaranth to a plate.

4. Add peeled and diced pear.

5. Mix yogurt with cocoa and add it to the plate. Sprinkle with cocoa.

BREAKFAST

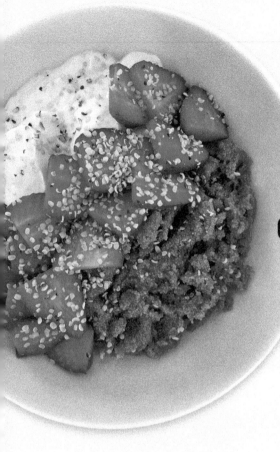

Amaranth With Yogurt & Strawberries

Visual Recipe by DAREBEE

© darebee.com

	SMALL	MEDIUM	LARGE
amaranth	⅓ cup ~ 70g	½ cup ~ 100g	1 cup ~ 200g
plain yogurt	4oz ~ 120ml	6oz ~ 180ml	8oz ~ 240ml
strawberries	4	6	8

LEVEL UP! Add hemp hearts.

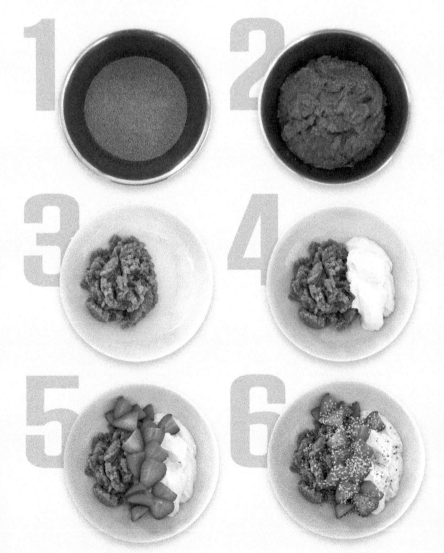

INSTRUCTIONS

1. Add amaranth to a cooking pot. Cover amaranth with double the amount of water and season for taste.

2. Bring water to a boil then lower heat to low. Cover the pot with a lid and simmer until it has completely absorbed the water ~ 15 minutes. The amaranth is cooked when it's no longer crunchy.

3. Transfer cooked amaranth to a plate.

4. Add yogurt.

5. Top with washed and sliced strawberries.

6. Sprinkle with hemp hearts.

BREAKFAST

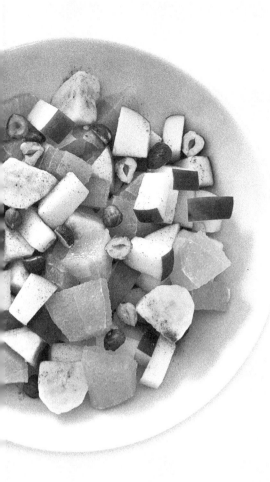

Apple & Orange Fruit Salad

Visual Recipe by DAREBEE
© darebee.com

	SMALL	MEDIUM	LARGE
apple	1	2	3
orange	1	2	2

LEVEL UP! Add banana, cinnamon and hazelnuts.

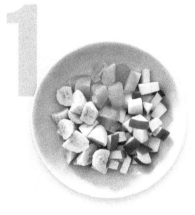
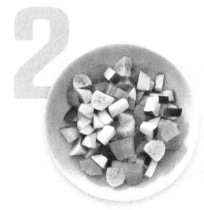
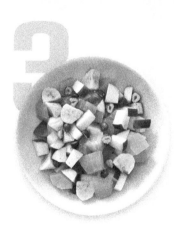

INSTRUCTIONS

1. Wash oranges and apples. Peel the oranges and cut all the fruit into bite-sized pieces. Reserve some of the orange.

2. Squeeze the reserved orange over the fruit and mix everything together.

3. Sprinkle with cinnamon and garnish with chopped hazelnuts, if using.

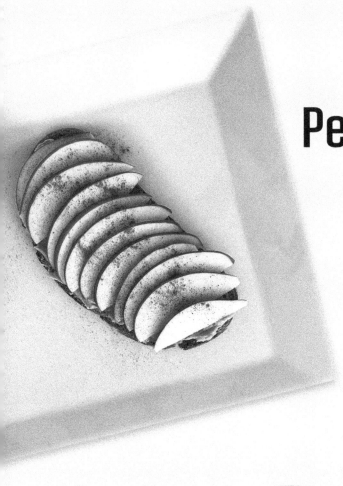

Apple Peanut Butter Toast

Visual Recipe
by DAREBEE
© darebee.com

	SMALL	MEDIUM	LARGE
bread	1 slice	2 slices	3 slices
apple	1	1	1
peanut butter	2 tbsps	4 tbsps	6 tbsps

LEVEL UP! Add cinnamon.

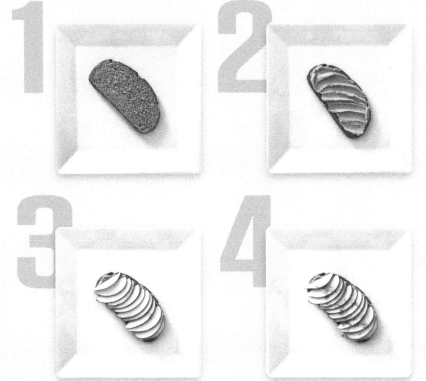

INSTRUCTIONS

1. Toast the bread.

2. Spread the peanut butter over the toast.

3. Slice the apple and arrange the slices on top of the toast.

4. Sprinkle with cinnamon.

BREAKFAST

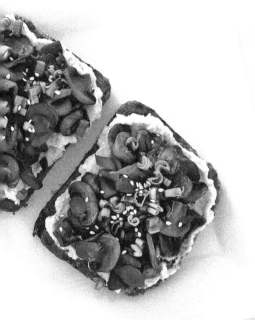

Avocado Mushroom Toast

**Visual Recipe
by DAREBEE
© darebee.com**

	SMALL	MEDIUM	LARGE
mushrooms	3oz ~ 90g	4oz ~ 120g	7oz ~ 200g
bread	1 slice	2 slices	3 slices
avocado	¼	⅓	½

LEVEL UP! Add fresh spring onions and sesame seeds.

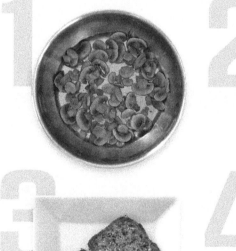
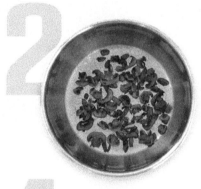

INSTRUCTIONS

1. Add mushrooms and ½ cup of water to a frying pan. Bring to a boil and cook on high heat until all the water has evaporated. Tip: You can use fresh or canned mushrooms.

2. Reduce heat to medium. Season for taste and stir continuously until the mushrooms become golden brown and begin to crisp at the edges.

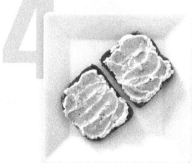

3. Toast the bread.

4. Cut, de-stone and peel the avocado. Mash it with a fork and spread on the toast.

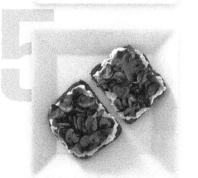
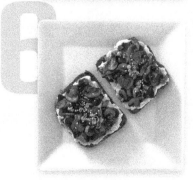

5. Add cooked mushrooms.

6. Garnish with spring onions and sesame seeds.

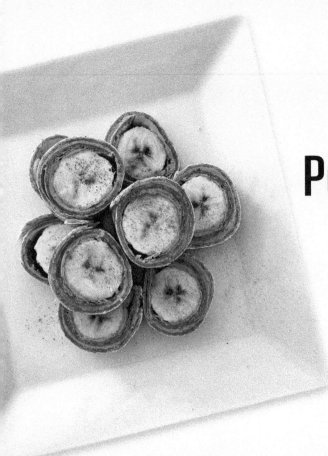

Banana Peanut Butter Rolls

Visual Recipe
by DAREBEE
© darebee.com

	SMALL	MEDIUM	LARGE
banana	1	1	2
tortilla wrap	1	1	2
peanut butter	1 tbsp	2 tbsps	4 tbsps

LEVEL UP! Add cinnamon.

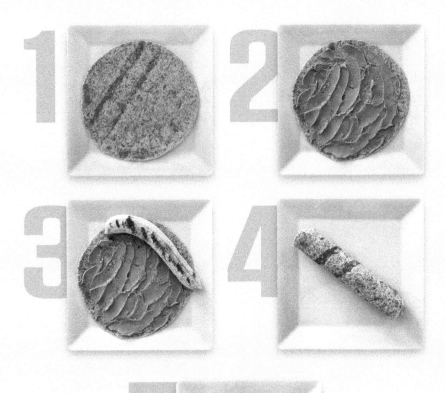

INSTRUCTIONS

1. Toast tortilla in the oven for 2 minutes.

2. Spread peanut butter over the tortilla.

3. Add ripe banana and sprinkle with cinnamon, if using.

4. Roll it up.

5. Cut into two or into bite-sized rolls and sprinkle with cinnamon again.

BREAKFAST

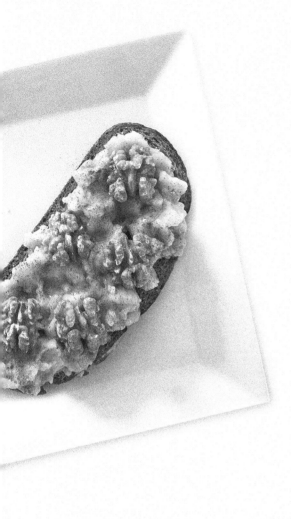

Banana Toast

Visual Recipe
by DAREBEE
© darebee.com

	SMALL	MEDIUM	LARGE
bread	1 slice	2 slices	3 slices
banana	1	2	3

LEVEL UP! Add walnuts and cinnamon.

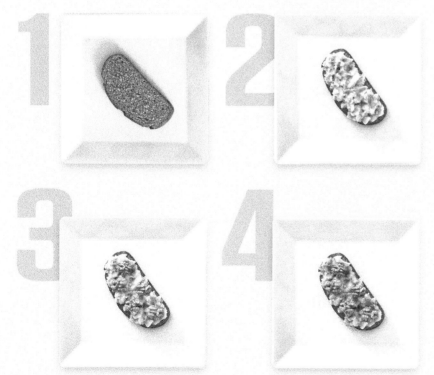

INSTRUCTIONS

1. Toast the bread.

2. Mash the banana with a fork and spread it over the toast.

3. Add walnuts.

4. Sprinkle with cinnamon.

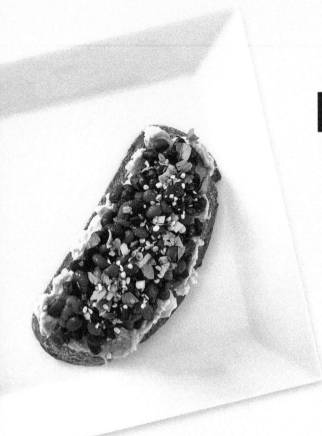

Black Bean Avocado Toast

Visual Recipe
by DAREBEE
© darebee.com

	SMALL	MEDIUM	LARGE
black beans	¼ cup ~ 50g	½ cup ~ 100g	1 cup ~ 200g
bread	1 slice	2 slices	3 slices
avocado	¼	⅓	½

LEVEL UP! Add parsley and hemp hearts.

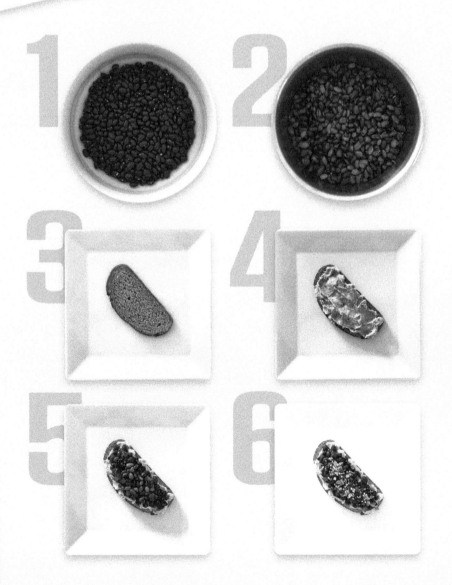

INSTRUCTIONS

1. Soak beans in plenty of water overnight. The next day, rinse and drain them.

2. Place the beans in a large cooking pot and cover with plenty of fresh water. Bring water to a boil then lower heat to low. Cover the pot with a lid. Simmer the beans until tender ~ 45-60 minutes. Drain. Alternatively, use canned beans: 1 can of cooked beans ~ 1 cup dry.

3. Toast the bread.

4. Cut, de-stone and peel the avocado. Mash it with a fork and spread on the toast.

5. Add black beans and season for taste.

6. Garnish with parsley and hemp hearts.

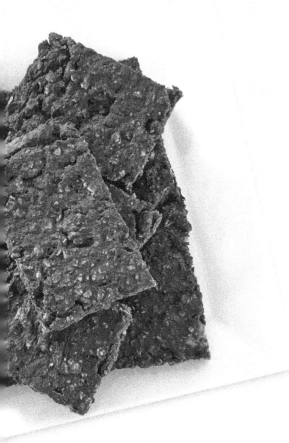

Black Bean Brownies

Visual Recipe
by DAREBEE
© darebee.com

	SMALL	MEDIUM	LARGE
black beans	¼ cup ~ 50g	½ cup ~ 100g	1 cup ~ 200g
oat flakes	¼ cup ~ 25g	½ cup ~ 50g	1 cup ~ 100g
cocoa	1 tbsp ~ 10g	2 tbsps ~ 20g	3 tbsps ~ 30g
milk	¼ cup ~ 50ml	½ cup ~ 100ml	1 cup ~ 200ml
banana	1 small	1	2

LEVEL UP! Add 1 teaspoon of baking powder to the mix.

INSTRUCTIONS

1. Soak beans in plenty of water overnight. The next day, rinse and drain them.

2. Place the beans in a large cooking pot and cover with plenty of fresh water. Bring water to a boil then lower heat to low. Cover the pot with a lid. Simmer the beans until tender ~ 45-60 minutes. Drain. Alternatively, use canned beans: 1 can of cooked beans ~ 1 cup dry.

3. Combine all of the ingredients in a mixing bowl.

4. Mash everything together with a potato masher, a spoon or a hand blender. If you want your brownies to be less chunky, blend until the batter is smooth. Add salt for taste or skip it.

5. Transfer the batter to a baking dish lined with baking paper and spread it with a spoon.

6. Preheat the oven to 400°F (200°C) and bake the brownies in the middle of the oven for 40 minutes. Let them rest for 30 minutes outside of the oven before cutting. Cut and serve.

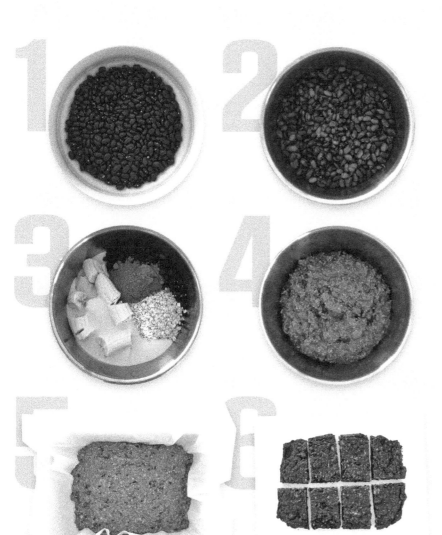

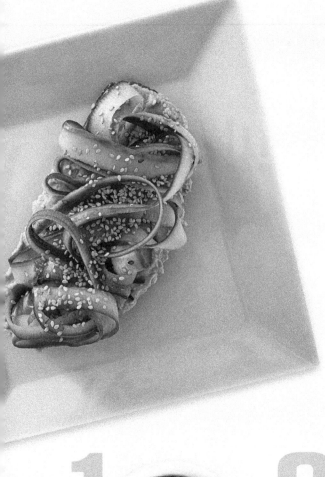

Chickpea Cucumber Toast

Visual Recipe by DAREBEE

© darebee.com

	SMALL	MEDIUM	LARGE
chickpeas	¼ cup ~ 50g	½ cup ~ 100g	1 cup ~ 200g
bread	1 slice	2 slices	3 slices
cucumber	1	1	2
tahini	½ tbsp	1 tbsp	2 tbsps

LEVEL UP! Add fresh garlic (or garlic powder) and sesame seeds.

INSTRUCTIONS

1. Soak chickpeas in plenty of water overnight. The next day, rinse and drain them.

2. Place chickpeas in a cooking pot and cover with plenty of fresh water. Bring water to a boil then lower heat to low. Cover the pot with a lid and simmer chickpeas for 30 minutes. They are cooked when tender. Drain. Alternatively, use canned chickpeas: 1 can of cooked chickpeas ~ 1 cup dry.

3. Drain the chickpeas and transfer to a bowl. Add garlic, tahini and ½ cup of water. Crush garlic, if using fresh.

4. Season for taste and mash chickpeas and tahini together with a fork until combined. Alternatively, blend in a blender until smooth.

5. Toast the bread and spread chickpea paste over a slice of bread.

6. Use a potato peeler to cut cucumber into ribbons and place on top of the toast. Sprinkle with sesame seeds.

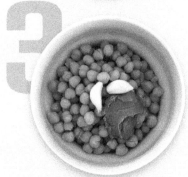
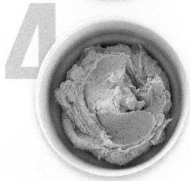
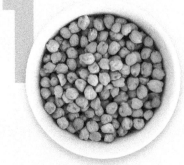
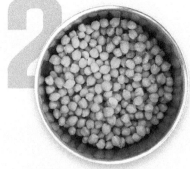
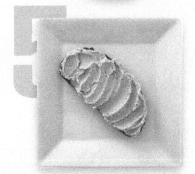
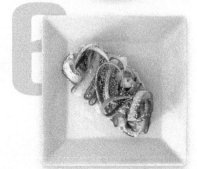

BREAKFAST

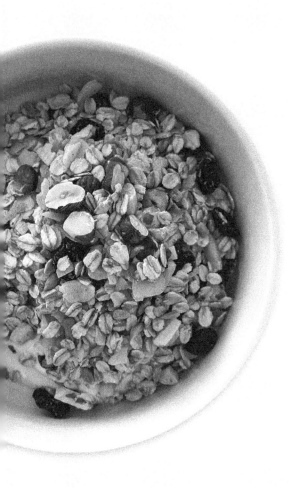

Granola With Yogurt

Visual Recipe
by DAREBEE
© darebee.com

	SMALL	MEDIUM	LARGE
rolled oats	½ cup ~ 50g	1 cup ~ 100g	1 ½ cup ~ 150g
butter	½ tbsp	1 tbsp	2 tbsps
plain yogurt	5oz ~ 150ml	7oz ~ 200ml	13oz ~ 400ml

LEVEL UP! Add sunflower seeds, coconut flakes, cranberries, hazelnuts.

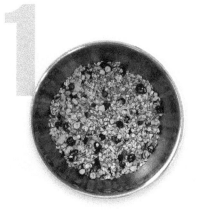
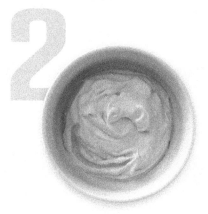
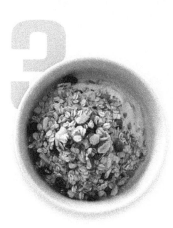

INSTRUCTIONS

1. Add butter to a frying pan. Heat it up and add rolled oats. Add any dried berries or dried fruit of your choice, nuts and seeds. Toast the oats for 5 minutes or until they begin to turn golden brown.

2. Transfer plain yogurt to a bowl.

3. Top with toasted oats.

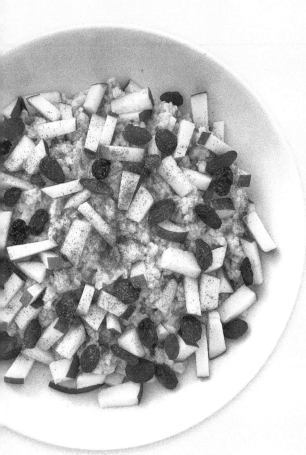

Oatmeal With Apple & Raisins

Visual Recipe
by DAREBEE
© darebee.com

	SMALL	MEDIUM	LARGE
oat flakes	½ cup ~ 50g	1 cup ~ 100g	1 ½ cup ~ 150g
apple	1	1	2
raisins	1oz ~ 30g	2oz ~ 60g	3oz ~ 90g

LEVEL UP! Add cinnamon and nutmeg.

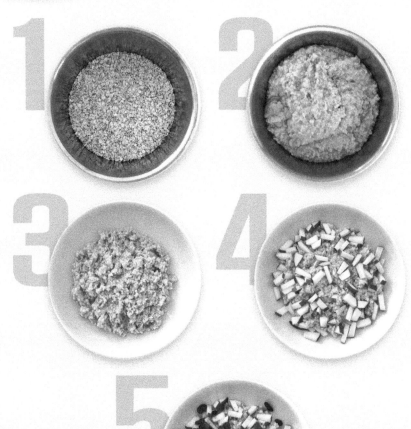

INSTRUCTIONS

1. Cover oat flakes with double the amount of water.

2. Bring to a boil and stir for 3 minutes until it thickens.

3. Transfer cooked oatmeal to a plate.

4. Add diced apple.

5. Add raisins and sprinkle with cinnamon and nutmeg.

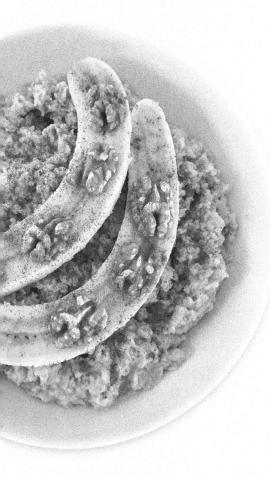

Oatmeal With Banana

Visual Recipe
by DAREBEE
© darebee.com

	SMALL	MEDIUM	LARGE
oat flakes	½ cup ~ 50g	1 cup ~ 100g	1 ½ cup ~ 150g
banana	1	1	2

LEVEL UP! Add walnuts and cinnamon.

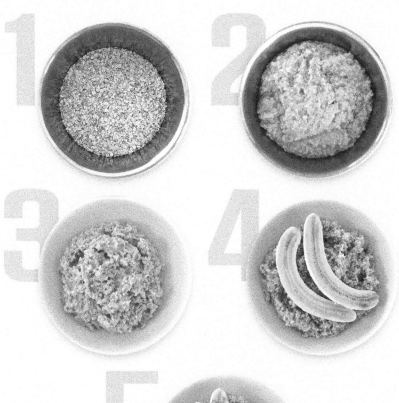

INSTRUCTIONS

1. Cover oat flakes with double the amount of water.

2. Bring to a boil and stir for 3 minutes or until it thickens.

3. Transfer cooked oatmeal to a plate.

4. Add banana sliced lengthwise.

5. Add walnuts and sprinkle with cinnamon.

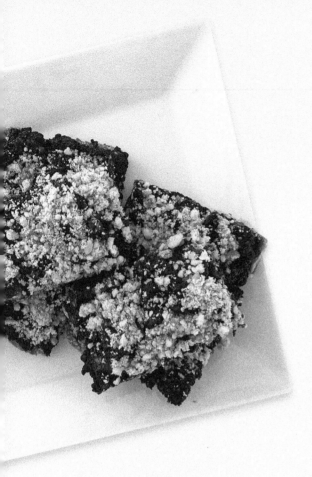

Oatmeal Blueberry Bake

Visual Recipe
by DAREBEE
© darebee.com

	SMALL	MEDIUM	LARGE
oat flakes	½ cup ~ 50g	1 cup ~ 100g	1 ½ cup ~ 150g
blueberries	½ cup ~ 70g	1 cup ~ 140g	1 ½ cup ~ 200g
maple syrup	1 tbsp	2 tbsps	3 tbsps

LEVEL UP! Add crushed walnuts and powdered clove.

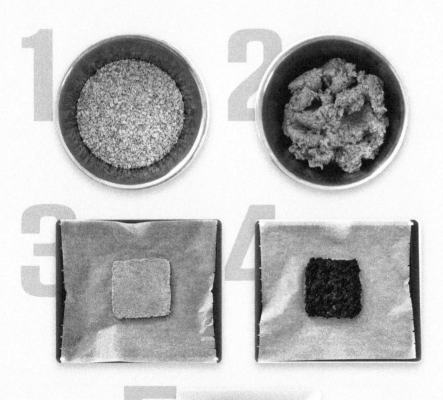

INSTRUCTIONS

1. Combine oat flakes and water 1:1 ratio in a cooking pot. Add maple or date serum and mix well.

2. Transfer to a cooking plate and bring to a boil. Stir for 2 minutes until the oatmeal mix thickens.

3. Split the mix into two halves. Transfer one half to a baking tray lined with baking paper and spread it with a spoon.

4. Mix the other half of the oatmeal with fresh or defrosted blueberries and spread it over the base.

5. Preheat the oven to 400ºF (200ºC). Bake in the oven for 30 minutes or until the crust becomes golden brown.

Sprinkle with powdered clove and top with crushed walnuts.

BREAKFAST

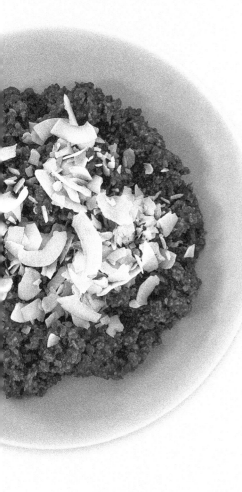

Chocolate Oatmeal With Coconut

Visual Recipe by DAREBEE
© darebee.com

	SMALL	MEDIUM	LARGE
oat flakes	½ cup ~ 50g	1 cup ~ 100g	1 ½ cup ~ 150g
cocoa	½ tbsp	1 tbsp	1 ½ tbsp
coconut flakes	1 tbsp	2 tbsps	3 tbsps

LEVEL UP! Use carob flour instead of cocoa powder.

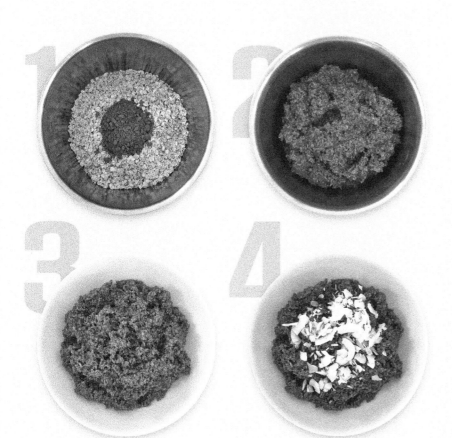

INSTRUCTIONS

1. Add oat flakes and cocoa powder to a cooking pot. Cover oat flakes with double the amount of water and mix.

2. Bring to a boil and stir for 3 minutes or until it thickens.

3. Transfer cooked oatmeal to a plate.

4. Top with coconut flakes.

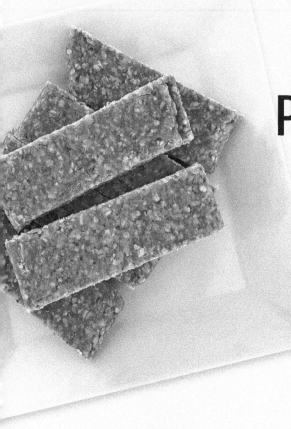

Oat Peanut Butter Bars

Visual Recipe by DAREBEE
© darebee.com

	SMALL	MEDIUM	LARGE
oat flakes	1 cup ~ 100g	2 cups ~ 200g	4 cups ~ 400g
peanut butter	2 tbsps ~ 40g	3 tbsps ~ 60g	4 tbsps ~ 80g
maple syrup	1 tbsp ~ 20ml	1 ½ tbsp ~ 30ml	2 tbsps ~ 40ml
water	¼ cup~ 50ml	½ cup ~ 100ml	1 cup ~ 200ml

LEVEL UP! Add crushed walnuts and dried cranberries to the mix.

INSTRUCTIONS

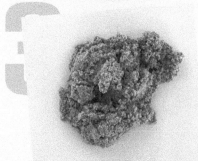
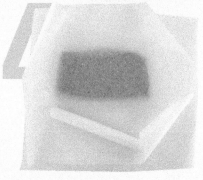

1. Add water, maple syrup and peanut butter to a large saucepan. Whisk together until combined. Alternatively, whisk together in a saucepan over medium heat.

2. Add oat flakes and mix until combined.

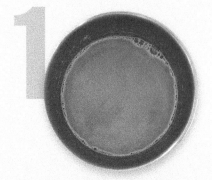
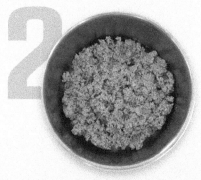

3. Transfer the mix to a countertop lined with baking paper. Cover with another sheet of baking paper and press down with a plate or roll it out using a rolling pin.

4. Lift the top sheet of baking paper off and fold the mix, cover back up and roll again until you get a thick rectangle.

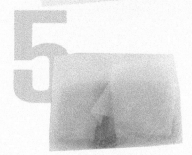
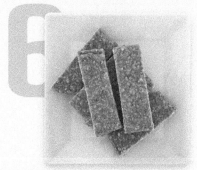

5. Wrap it up and place into the fridge to chill overnight or for a minimum of 4 hours.

6. The next day take it out and cut into bars.

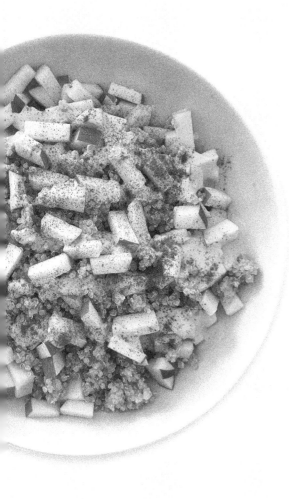

Quinoa With Apple & Peanut Sauce

Visual Recipe
by DAREBEE
© darebee.com

	SMALL	MEDIUM	LARGE
quinoa	⅓ cup ~ 70g	½ cup ~ 100g	1 cup ~ 200g
apple	1	1	2
peanut butter	1 tbsp	1 ½ tbsp	2 tbsps

LEVEL UP! Add cinnamon.

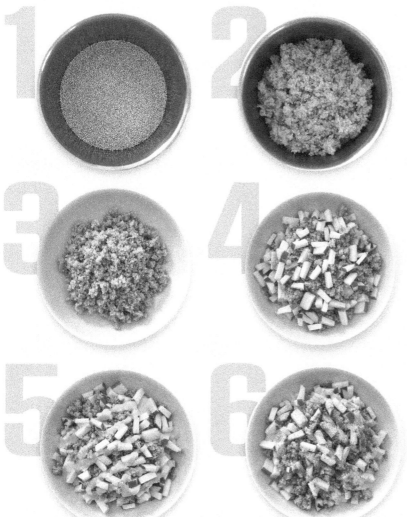

INSTRUCTIONS

1. Rinse quinoa really well until the water runs clear.

2. Transfer the quinoa to a cooking pot. Cover with double the amount of water and stir once. Bring water to a boil then lower heat to low. Cover with a lid. Cook the quinoa until it is tender and it has completely absorbed the water ~ 15 minutes.

3. Transfer cooked quinoa to a plate.

4. Add sliced apple.

5. Combine peanut butter with water 1:3 ratio and stir until creamy. Drizzle over the quinoa.

6. Sprinkle with cinnamon.

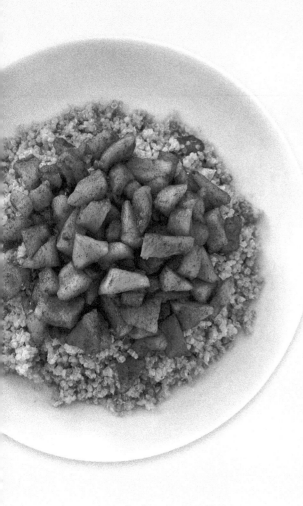

Quinoa With Spiced Apple

Visual Recipe
by DAREBEE
© darebee.com

	SMALL	MEDIUM	LARGE
quinoa	⅓ cup ~ 70g	½ cup ~ 100g	1 cup ~ 200g
apple	1	2	3
cinnamon	½ tsp	1 tsp	1 ½ tsp

LEVEL UP! Add a pinch of nutmeg and clove to the apples.

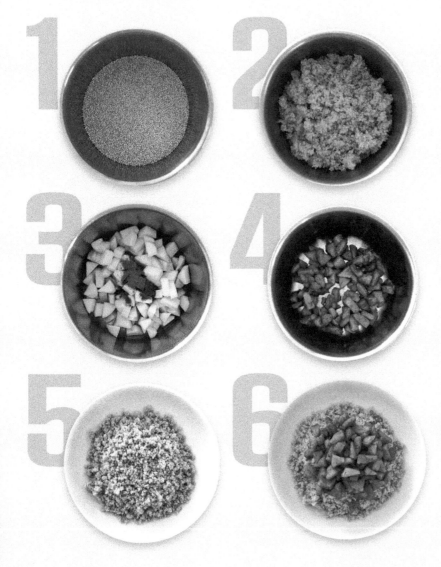

INSTRUCTIONS

1. Rinse quinoa really well.

2. Transfer the quinoa to a cooking pot. Cover with double the amount of water and stir once. Bring water to a boil then lower heat to low. Cover with a lid. Cook the quinoa until it is tender and it has completely absorbed the water ~ 15 minutes.

3. In the meantime, peel and dice the apples. Add them to a saucepan with ½ cup of water. Add spices and mix.

4. Bring water to a boil then lower heat to medium. Cover with a lid and set a timer 10 minutes or until all the water has evaporated.

5. Transfer cooked quinoa to a plate.

6. Top with spiced apples.

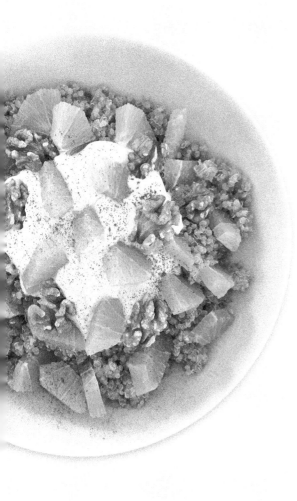

Quinoa With Yogurt & Orange

Visual Recipe
by DAREBEE
© darebee.com

	SMALL	MEDIUM	LARGE
quinoa	⅓ cup ~ 70g	½ cup ~ 100g	1 cup ~ 200g
plain yogurt	4oz ~ 120ml	6oz ~ 180ml	8oz ~ 240ml
orange	1	1	2

LEVEL UP! Add walnuts and cinnamon.

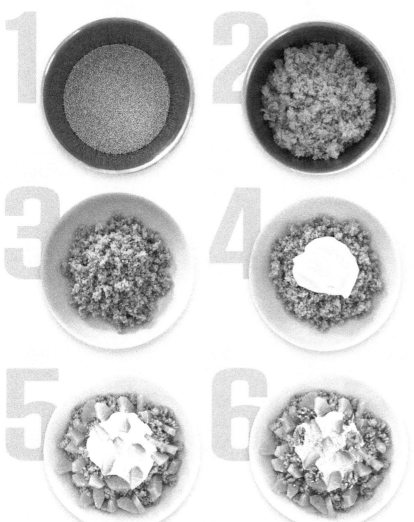

INSTRUCTIONS

1. Rinse quinoa really well until the water runs clear.

2. Transfer the quinoa to a cooking pot. Cover with double the amount of water and stir once. Bring water to a boil then lower heat to low. Cover with a lid. Cook the quinoa until it is tender and it has completely absorbed the water ~ 15 minutes.

3. Transfer cooked quinoa to a plate.

4. Add yogurt.

5. Add sliced orange.

6. Add walnuts and sprinkle with cinnamon.

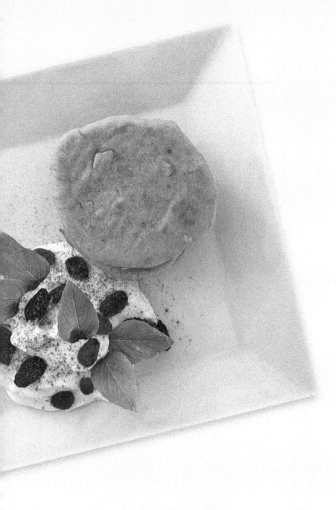

Sweet Potato Pancakes

Visual Recipe
by DAREBEE
© darebee.com

	SMALL	MEDIUM	LARGE
sweet potato	1 small ~ 120g	1 ~ 240g	2 ~ 480g
milk	4oz ~ 120ml	8oz ~ 240ml	16oz ~ 480ml
flour	2oz ~ 60g	4oz ~ 120g	7oz ~ 240g

LEVEL UP! Add 1 tsp of baking powder to the batter. Add yogurt, raisins, fresh basil and nutmeg.

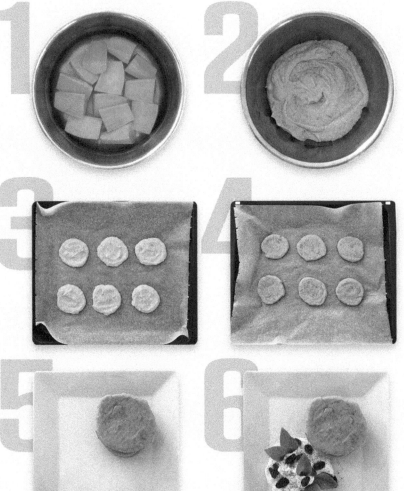

INSTRUCTIONS

1. Add peeled and cut sweet potato to a cooking pot and cover with water. Bring water to a boil then lower heat to low. Simmer for 15 minutes or until the potatoes are soft all the way through.

2. Drain the potatoes. Add milk, flour and baking powder. Mix until smooth.

3. Spoon equal portions of the batter to a baking tray lined with baking paper. Spread to form pancakes.

4. Preheat the oven to 400ºF (200ºC). Bake the pancakes for 10 minutes. Flip them over and bake for another 10 minutes or until the crust begins to turn golden brown. Alternatively, fry in a non-stick frying pan for 3 minutes on each side.

5. Transfer the pancakes to a plate and place on top of each other.

6. Garnish with yogurt, fresh basil and raisins. Sprinkle with nutmeg.

BREAKFAST

White Bean Tomato Toast

Visual Recipe by DAREBEE
© darebee.com

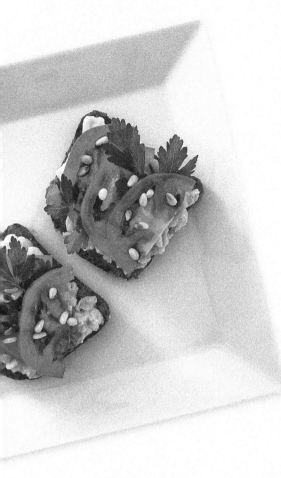

	SMALL	MEDIUM	LARGE
white beans	¼ cup ~ 50g	½ cup ~ 100g	1 cup ~ 200g
bread	1 slice	2 slices	3 slices
tomato	1	1	1

LEVEL UP! Add balsamic vinegar, fresh parsley and pine nuts.

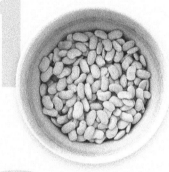
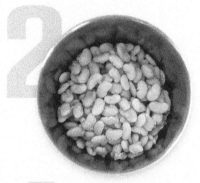
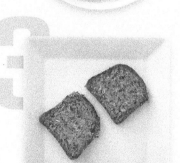
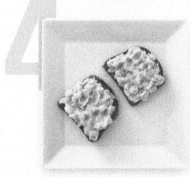
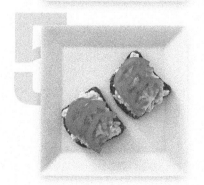
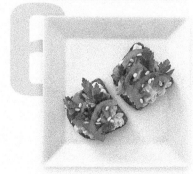

INSTRUCTIONS

1. Soak beans in plenty of water overnight. The next day, rinse and drain them.

2. Place the beans in a large cooking pot and cover with plenty of fresh water. Bring water to a boil then lower heat to low. Cover the pot with a lid. Simmer the beans until tender ~ 30 minutes. Drain. Alternatively, use canned beans: 1 can of cooked beans ~ 1 cup dry.

3. Toast the bread.

4. Season for taste and mash the beans. Spread them on top of the toast.

5. Add sliced tomatoes.

6. Top with parsley and pine nuts. Drizzle with balsamic vinegar or balsamic sauce.

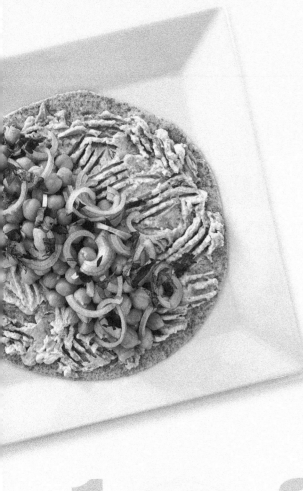

Avocado Chickpea Tortilla Wrap

Visual Recipe by DAREBEE
© darebee.com

	SMALL	MEDIUM	LARGE
chickpeas	¼ cup ~ 50g	½ cup ~ 100g	1 cup ~ 200g
tortilla wrap	1	1	2
avocado	¼	½	1

LEVEL UP! Add red onion and sesame seeds.

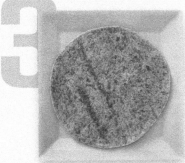
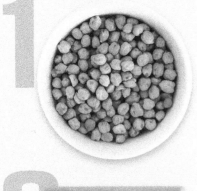
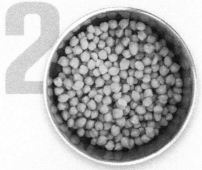
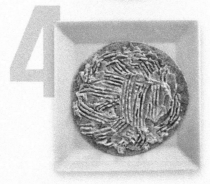
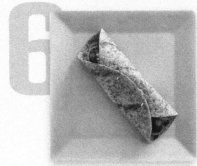
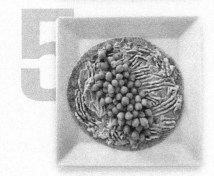

INSTRUCTIONS

1. Soak chickpeas in plenty of water overnight. The next day, rinse and drain them.

2. Place chickpeas in a cooking pot and cover with plenty of fresh water. Bring water to a boil then lower heat to low. Cover the pot with a lid and simmer chickpeas for 30 minutes. They are cooked when tender. Drain. Alternatively, use canned chickpeas: 1 can of cooked chickpeas ~ 1 cup dry.

3. Toast tortilla in the oven for 2 minutes.

4. Cut, de-stone and peel the avocado. Mash it with a fork and spread on the tortilla.

5. Add chickpeas and season for taste.

6. Garnish with red onion and sesame seeds. Fold it up.

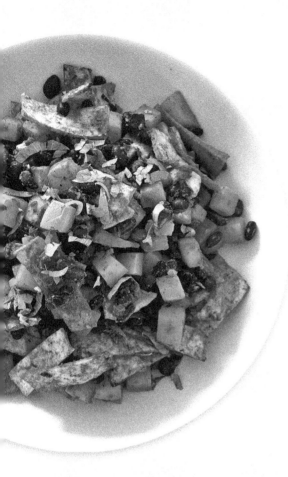

Black Bean Butternut Squash Enchiladas

Visual Recipe by DAREBEE
© darebee.com

	SMALL	MEDIUM	LARGE
black beans	¼ cup ~ 50g	½ cup ~ 100g	1 cup ~ 200g
butternut squash	7oz ~ 200g	10oz ~ 300g	12oz ~ 400g
tortilla	1	2	3
tomato paste	1 tbsp	2 tbsps	3 tbsps
molasses	1 tsp	2 tsps	3 tsps
water	¼ cup ~ 50ml	⅓ cup ~ 70ml	½ cup ~ 100ml

LEVEL UP! Add ½ tablespoon black pepper and ½ tablespoon cayenne pepper to the sauce for the extra kick.

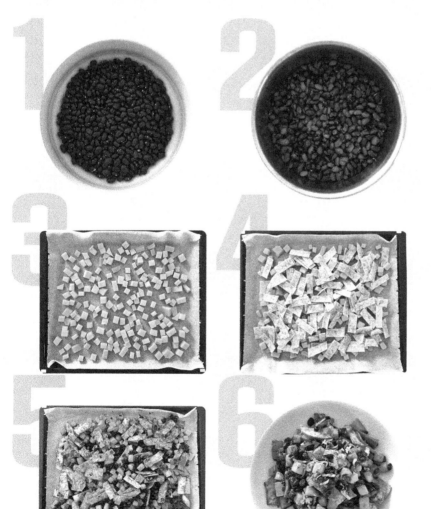

INSTRUCTIONS

1. Soak beans in plenty of water overnight. The next day, rinse and drain them.

2. Place the beans in a large cooking pot and cover with plenty of fresh water. Bring water to a boil then lower heat to low. Cover the pot with a lid. Simmer the beans until tender ~ 45-60 minutes. Drain. Alternatively, use canned beans: 1 can of cooked beans ~ 1 cup dry.

3. Peel and dice butternut squash. Transfer to a baking tray lined with baking paper and arrange in a single layer. Season for taste. Preheat the oven to 400°F (200°C). Roast butternut squash in the middle of the oven for 10 minutes or until it's soft all the way through.

4. Cut the tortilla into strips and arrange them on top of the butternut squash.

5. Mix tomato paste, molasses and water together to make the sauce then combine it with the drained beans. Add the beans to the butternut squash and tortilla strips and toss everything together until well coated. Bake in the middle of the oven for 15 minutes or until tortilla strips begin to crisp up.

6. Transfer to a plate and garnish with fresh parsley.

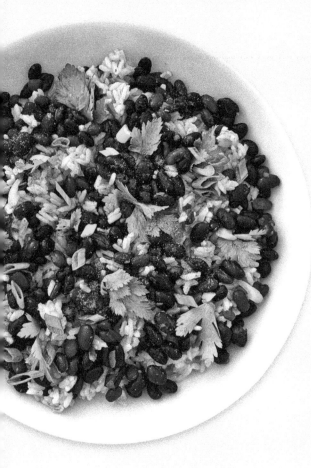

Black Beans With Rice

Visual Recipe
by DAREBEE
© darebee.com

	SMALL	MEDIUM	LARGE
black beans	¼ cup ~ 50g	½ cup ~ 100g	1 cup ~ 200g
rice	¼ cup ~ 50g	⅓ cup ~ 70g	½ cup ~ 100g

LEVEL UP! Add parsley, spring onions and cumin.

INSTRUCTIONS

1. Soak beans in plenty of water overnight. The next day, rinse and drain them.

2. Place the beans in a large cooking pot and cover with plenty of fresh water. Bring water to a boil then lower heat to low. Cover the pot with a lid. Simmer the beans until tender ~ 45-60 minutes. Drain. Alternatively, use canned beans: 1 can of cooked beans ~ 1 cup dry.

3. Rinse rice really well.

4. Transfer the rice to a cooking pot. Cover with double the amount of water, season for taste and stir once. Bring water to a boil then lower heat to low. Cover with a lid and simmer until it has completely absorbed the water. It will take ~ 20 minutes for white rice; 35 minutes for brown rice.

5. Add cooked rice and cooked drained beans to a plate. Season for taste and mix together.

6. Garnish with parsley, spring onions and sprinkle with cumin.

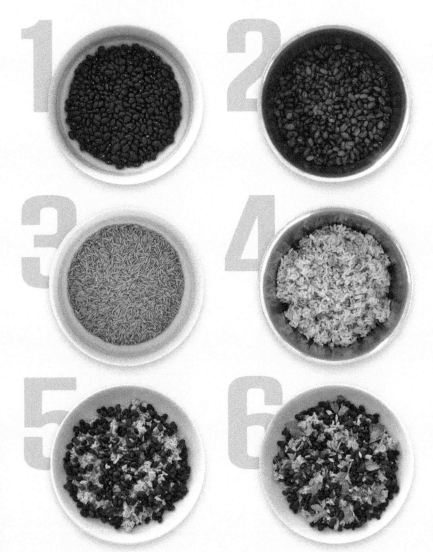

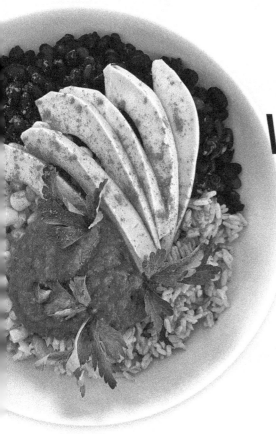

Black Beans With Rice, Corn & Avocado

Visual Recipe by DAREBEE
© darebee.com

	SMALL	MEDIUM	LARGE
black beans	¼ cup ~ 50g	½ cup ~ 100g	1 cup ~ 200g
rice	¼ cup ~ 50g	⅓ cup ~ 70g	½ cup ~ 100g
corn	¼ cup ~ 40g	¼ cup ~ 40g	½ cup ~ 80g
avocado	¼	⅓	½

LEVEL UP! Add ready salsa sauce, parsley and cayenne pepper.

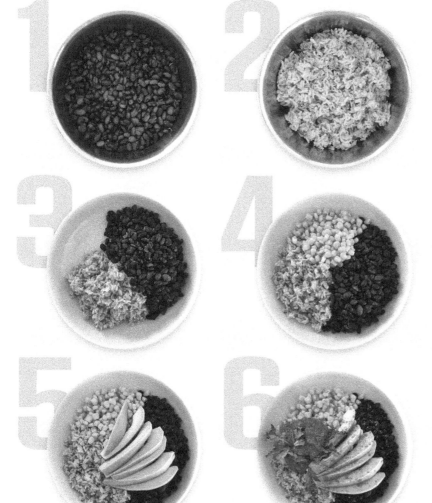

INSTRUCTIONS

1. Soak beans in plenty of water overnight. The next day, rinse and drain them. Place the beans in a large cooking pot and cover with plenty of fresh water. Bring water to a boil then lower heat to low. Cover the pot with a lid. Simmer the beans until tender ~ 45-60 minutes. Drain. Alternatively, use canned beans: 1 can of cooked beans ~ 1 cup dry.

2. Rinse the rice really well until the water runs clear. Transfer the rice to a cooking pot. Cover with double the amount of water and stir once. Bring water to a boil then lower heat to low. Cover with a lid and set a timer: 20 minutes for white rice; 35 minutes for brown rice.

3. Add cooked rice and cooked drained beans to a plate.

4. Add sweet corn. If using frozen sweet corn, place it in a saucepan, cover with water and bring to a boil. Drain.

5. Add sliced avocado and season for taste.

6. Add salsa, top with parsley and sprinkle with cayenne pepper.

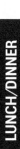

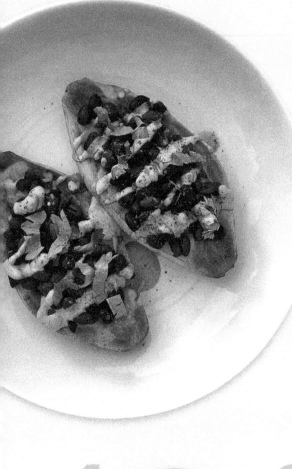

Black Bean Stuffed Sweet Potato

Visual Recipe by DAREBEE © darebee.com

	SMALL	MEDIUM	LARGE
black beans	¼ cup ~ 50g	½ cup ~ 100g	1 cup ~ 200g
sweet potato	1 small	1	2
tahini	½ tbsp	1 tbsp	2 tbsps

LEVEL UP! Add fresh parsley and cumin.

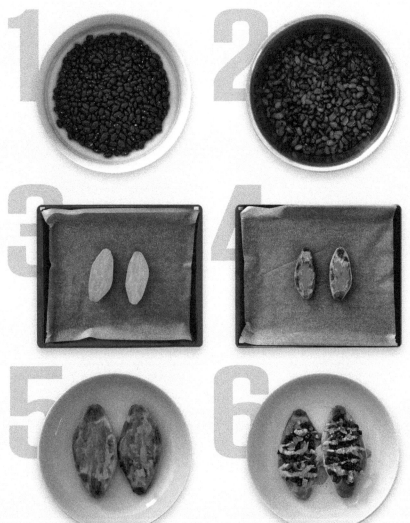

INSTRUCTIONS

1. Soak beans in plenty of water overnight. The next day, rinse and drain them.

2. Place the beans in a large cooking pot and cover with plenty of fresh water. Bring water to a boil then lower heat to low. Cover the pot with a lid. Simmer the beans until tender ~ 45-60 minutes. Drain. Alternatively, use canned beans: 1 can of cooked beans ~ 1 cup dry.

3. Peel sweet potato, cut it in half and transfer to a baking tray lined with baking paper.

4. Preheat the oven to 400°F (200°C). Bake the potatoes in the oven for 30 minutes or until tender.

5. Transfer the potato to a plate and use a fork to make a well in the middle.

6. Add cooked beans and season for taste. Top with tahini thinned with water 1:3 and parsley. Sprinkle with cumin.

LUNCH/DINNER

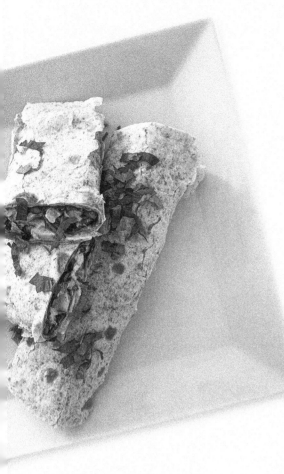

Black Bean Tortilla Wrap

Visual Recipe
by DAREBEE
© darebee.com

	SMALL	MEDIUM	LARGE
black beans	¼ cup ~ 50g	½ cup ~ 100g	1 cup ~ 200g
tortilla wrap	1	1	2
cucumber	1	1	2
plain yogurt	2oz ~ 60ml	3oz ~ 90ml	4oz ~ 120ml

LEVEL UP! Add fresh parsley, cumin and garlic powder.

INSTRUCTIONS

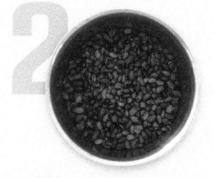
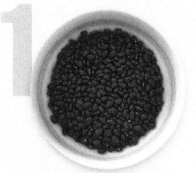
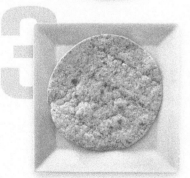
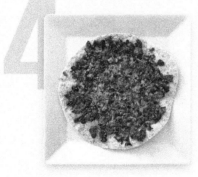
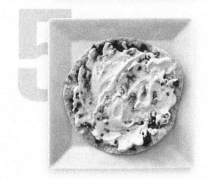
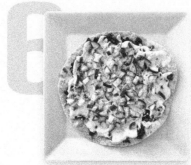

1. Soak beans in plenty of water overnight. The next day, rinse and drain them.

2. Place the beans in a large cooking pot and cover with plenty of fresh water. Bring water to a boil then lower heat to low. Cover the pot with a lid. Simmer the beans until tender ~ 45-60 minutes. Drain. Alternatively, use canned beans: 1 can of cooked beans ~ 1 cup dry.

3. Toast tortilla in the oven for 2 minutes.

4. Fill a tortilla wrap with beans and mash them with a fork.

5. Mix yogurt with cumin and garlic powder and spread it over the beans.

6. Add diced cucumber, season for taste and fold into a roll. Garnish with parsley.

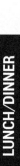

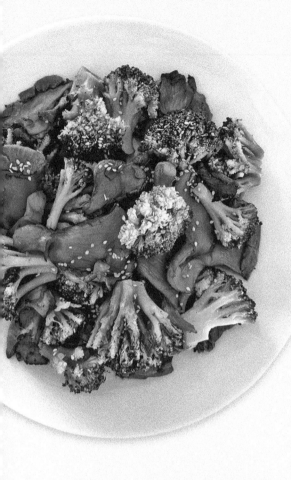

Broccoli With Mushrooms

Visual Recipe
by DAREBEE
© darebee.com

	SMALL	MEDIUM	LARGE
broccoli	1 cup ~ 150g	2 cups ~ 300g	2 cups ~ 300g
mushrooms	7oz ~ 200g	10oz ~ 300g	13oz ~ 400g
balsamic vinegar	1 tbsp	2 tbsps	3 tbsps

LEVEL UP! Add soy sauce and sesame seeds.

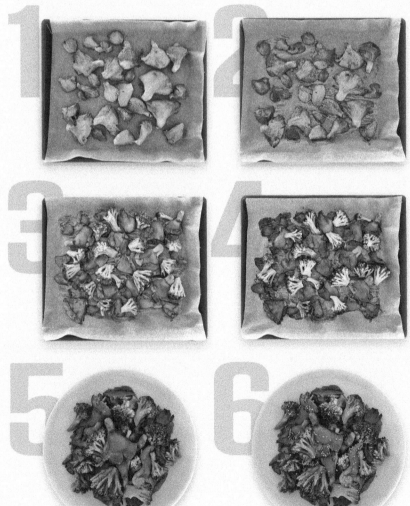

INSTRUCTIONS

1. Clean mushrooms and coat them in balsamic vinegar. Arrange them on top of a baking tray lined with baking paper.

2. Preheat the oven to 400ºF (200ºC). Roast mushrooms in the middle of the oven for 20 minutes or until they begin to brown.

3. Take the mushrooms out of the oven, flip them over and add broccoli florets. Drizzle with soy sauce, season for taste and place back into the oven. The florets can be taken directly from the freezer.

4. Place the tray back into the oven and roast the mushrooms and the broccoli for another 10 minutes.

5. Transfer mushroom and broccoli to a plate.

6. Sprinkle with sesame seeds.

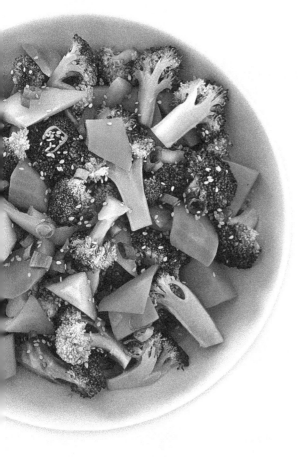

Broccoli Stir-Fry

Visual Recipe
by DAREBEE
© darebee.com

	SMALL	MEDIUM	LARGE
broccoli	1 cup ~ 150g	2 cups ~ 300g	3 cups ~ 450g
carrots	1	1	2
bell pepper	1	1	2
sesame oil	½ tbsp	½ tbsp	1 tbsp

LEVEL UP! Add fresh garlic, spring onions and sesame seeds.

INSTRUCTIONS

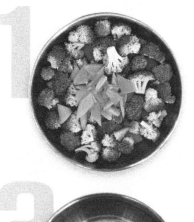
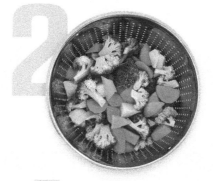

1. Split broccoli into bite-sized florets. Peel the carrot and de-seed the bell pepper. Cut both into bite-sized pieces. Fill a large pan with water and bring it to a boil. Add carrots. Set the timer to 7 minutes. Two minutes in, add broccoli. Five minutes in, add bell pepper.

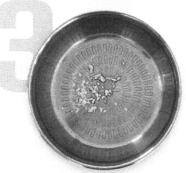
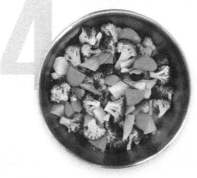

2. Remove from heat, transfer the vegetables into a colander and run under cold water under the tap to stop them from cooking any further.

3. Clean, finely dice garlic cloves, if using, and add them to a frying pan along with sesame oil. Set heat to high.

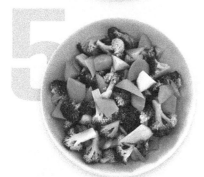
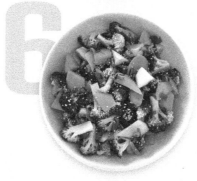

4. Once the frying pan heats up, add blanched vegetables and stir fry for 2 minutes. Season for taste and keep stirring.

5. Transfer to a plate.

6. Garnish with spring onions and sprinkle with sesame seeds. Serve with soy sauce and eat with chopsticks.

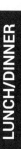

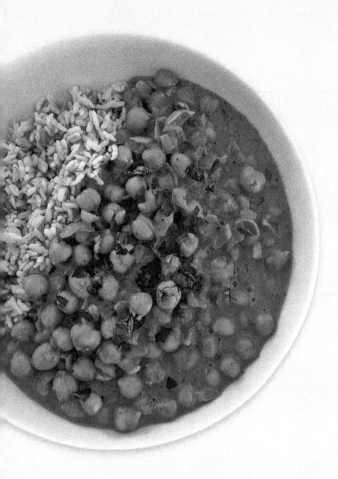

Chickpea Curry with Rice

Visual Recipe
by DAREBEE
© darebee.com

	SMALL	MEDIUM	LARGE
rice	¼ cup ~ 50g	⅓ cup ~ 70g	½ cup ~ 100g
chickpeas	¼ cup ~ 50g	½ cup ~ 100g	1 cup ~ 200g
onion	1	1	1
tomato	1	1	1
cooking cream	3oz ~ 100ml	5oz ~ 150ml	7oz ~ 200ml
molasses	1 tsp	2 tsps	3 tsps
curry powder	½ tbsp	1 tbsp	1 ½ tbsps

LEVEL UP! Add fresh parsley.

INSTRUCTIONS

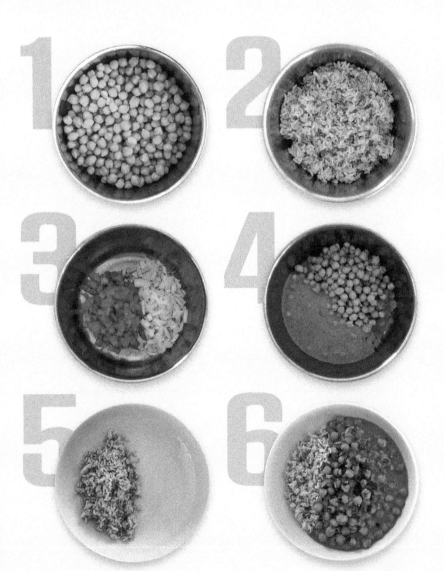

1. Soak chickpeas in plenty of water overnight. The next day, rinse and drain them. Place chickpeas in a cooking pot and cover with plenty of fresh water. Bring water to a boil then lower heat to low. Cover the pot with a lid and simmer chickpeas for 30 minutes. They are cooked when tender. Drain. Alternatively, use canned chickpeas: 1 can of cooked chickpeas ~ 1 cup dry.

2. Rinse the rice really well until the water runs clear. Transfer the rice to a cooking pot. Cover with double the amount of water and stir once. Bring water to a boil then lower heat to low. Cover with a lid and set a timer: 20 minutes for white rice; 35 minutes for brown rice.

3. Finely dice onion and tomato. Add to a cooking pot with ½ cup of water. Bring to a boil and reduce heat to medium. Saute until all the water has evaporated.

4. Combine cooking cream, molasses and curry powder together in a bowl and mix well. Add it and the chickpeas to the tomatoes and onions. Season for taste. Mix together and cook over medium heat for another 3-4 minutes.

5. Transfer rice to a plate.

6. Add chickpea curry and garnish with fresh parsley.

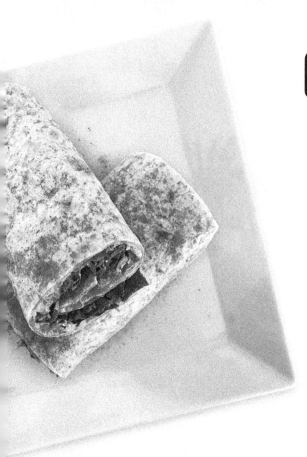

Chickpea Tortilla Wrap

Visual Recipe
by DAREBEE
© darebee.com

	SMALL	MEDIUM	LARGE
chickpeas	¼ cup ~ 50g	½ cup ~ 100g	1 cup ~ 200g
tortilla wrap	1	1	2
tahini	½ tbsp	1 tbsp	2 tbsps
lettuce	1 cup ~ 50g	1 cup ~ 50g	1 cup ~ 50g

LEVEL UP! Add fresh or powdered garlic and cayenne pepper.

INSTRUCTIONS

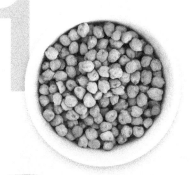
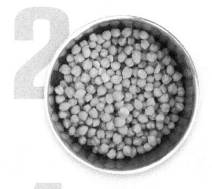

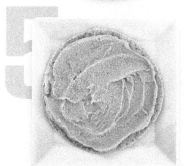
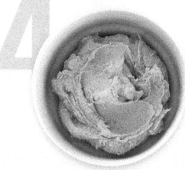

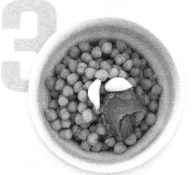
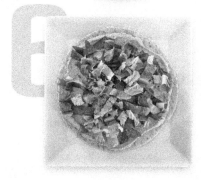

1. Soak chickpeas in plenty of water overnight. The next day, rinse and drain them.

2. Place chickpeas in a cooking pot and cover with plenty of fresh water. Bring water to a boil then lower heat to low. Cover the pot with a lid and simmer chickpeas for 30 minutes. They are cooked when tender. Drain. Alternatively, use canned chickpeas: 1 can of cooked chickpeas ~ 1 cup dry.

3. Transfer drained chickpeas to a bowl. Add garlic, tahini and ½ cup of water. Crush garlic, if using fresh.

4. Season for taste and mash chickpeas and tahini together with a fork until combined. Alternatively, blend in a blender until smooth.

5. Toast tortilla in the oven for 2 minutes then spread chickpea tahini paste on top of it.

6. Add chopped up lettuce, fold into a roll, cut into two halves and sprinkle with cayenne pepper.

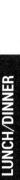

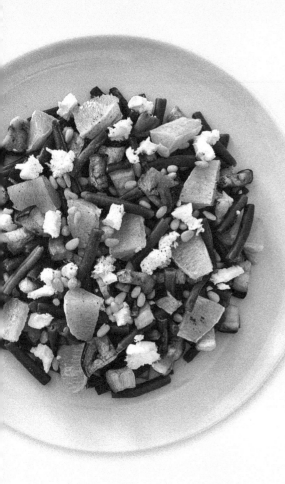

Eggplant & Green Beans With Oranges

Visual Recipe
by DAREBEE
© darebee.com

	SMALL	MEDIUM	LARGE
eggplant	1	2	3
green beans	1 cup	2 cups	3 cups
oranges	1	1	2

LEVEL UP! Add white cheese, pine nuts and black pepper.

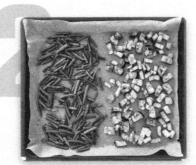
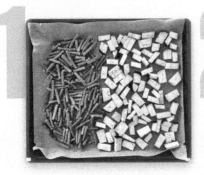
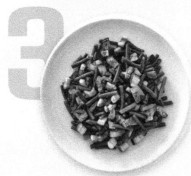
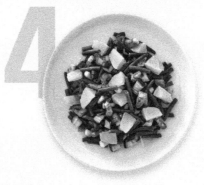
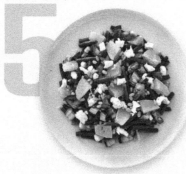

INSTRUCTIONS

1. Cut eggplant and green beans into bite-sized pieces and arrange them on top of a baking tray lined with baking paper.

2. Preheat the oven to 400°F (200°C). Roast eggplant and green beans in the oven for 15 minutes or until it begins to brown.

3. Transfer to a plate and season for taste.

4. Add cut orange. Squeeze some of the orange juice over the eggplant and beans.

5. Add crumbled white cheese. Top with pine nuts and sprinkle with black pepper.

LUNCH/DINNER

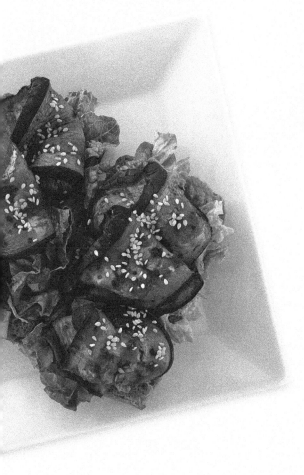

Eggplant Toast

Visual Recipe
by DAREBEE
© darebee.com

	SMALL	MEDIUM	LARGE
eggplant	1	2	3
bread	1 slice	2 slices	3 slices
lettuce	½ cup ~ 25g	1 cup~ 50g	1 cup~ 50g
tomato paste	1 tbsp	2 tbsps	3 tbsps
molasses	1 tsp	2 tsps	3 tsps
smoked paprika	1 tsp	1 ½ tsp	2 tsps

LEVEL UP! Add 1 tsp liquid smoke to the tomato mix. Add sesame seeds.

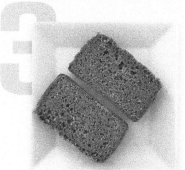
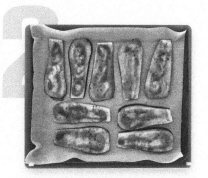
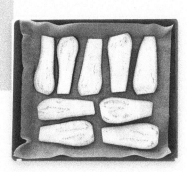
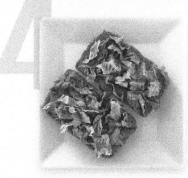
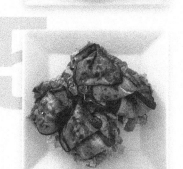
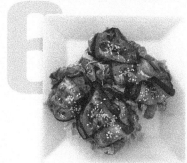

INSTRUCTIONS

1. Cut eggplant into thin slices lengthwise and arrange them on top of a baking tray lined with baking paper.

2. Combine tomato paste, molasses, smoked paprika and 1/2 cup of water and mix well. Add liquid smoke, if using, and season for taste. Coat both sides of the eggplant slices with the sauce. Preheat the oven to 400ºF (200ºC). Roast eggplant in the oven for 15-20 minutes or until it begins to brown.

3. Toast the bread.

4. Add cut lettuce.

5. Add cooked eggplant slices.

6. Top with sesame seeds.

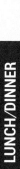

LUNCH/DINNER

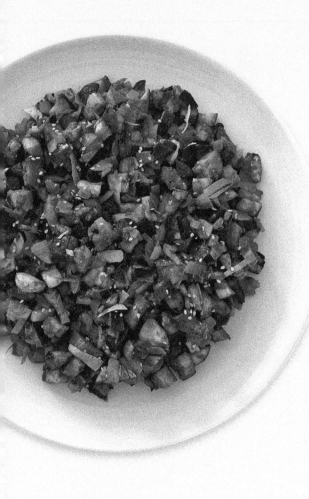

Eggplant & Zucchini In Tomato Sauce

Visual Recipe by DAREBEE
© darebee.com

	SMALL	MEDIUM	LARGE
eggplant	1	2	3
zucchini	1	2	3
onion	1	1	2
tomato sauce	½ cup ~ 100ml	1 cup ~ 200ml	1 ½ cup ~ 300ml

LEVEL UP! Add ½ tbsp cinnamon, fresh basil and sesame seeds.

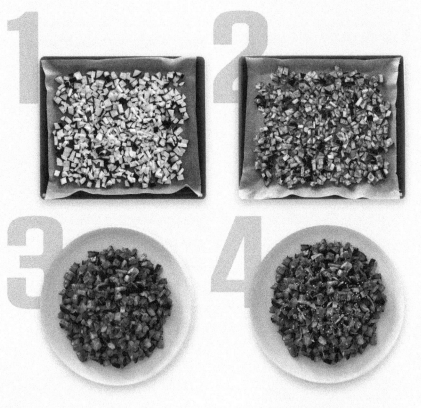

INSTRUCTIONS

1. Dice eggplant, zucchini and onion and arrange them on top of a baking tray lined with baking paper. Season for taste.

2. Sprinkle the vegetables with cinnamon, if using, and cover with tomato sauce. Mix well so all of the vegetables are coated. Preheat the oven to 400ºF (200ºC). Roast eggplant in the oven for 15-20 minutes or until it begins to brown.

3. Transfer to a plate.

4. Garnish with fresh basil and sesame seeds. It also goes well with white cheese.

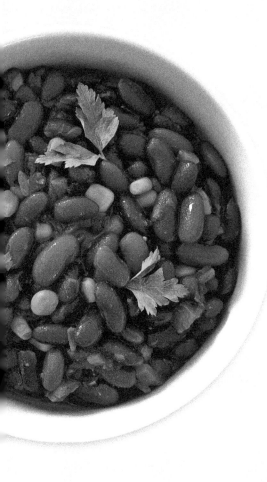

Kidney Bean Chili

Visual Recipe
by DAREBEE
© darebee.com

	SMALL	MEDIUM	LARGE
kidney beans	¼ cup ~ 50g	½ cup ~ 100g	1 cup ~ 200g
onion	1	2	2
corn	¼ cup ~ 40g	¼ cup ~ 40g	½ cup ~ 80g
bell pepper	1	1	1
tomato paste	1 tbsp	2 tbsps	3 tbsps
molasses	1 tsp	2 tsps	3 tsps
chili powder	1 tsp	1 ½ tsp	2 tsps

LEVEL UP! Add spring onions.

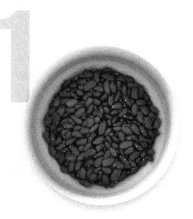
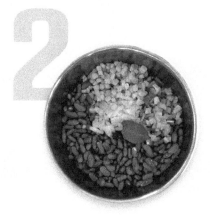
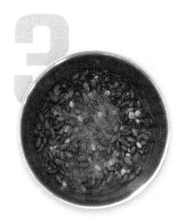

INSTRUCTIONS

1. Soak kidney beans in plenty of water overnight. The next day, rinse and drain them. Alternatively, use canned beans: 1 can of cooked kidney beans ~ 1 cup dry.

2. Dice onion and green bell pepper. Combine all of the ingredients in a large cooking pot and season for taste. You can take corn directly from the freezer. Bring to a boil, lower the heat to low, cover the pot with a lid and let simmer for: 30 minutes, if using canned beans; 45 minutes, if using soaked beans.

3. Garnish with spring onions.

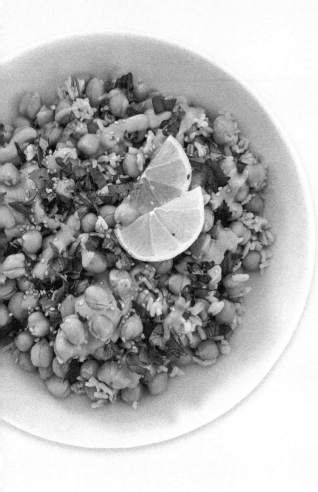

Lemon Chickpea Rice

Visual Recipe
by DAREBEE
© darebee.com

	SMALL	MEDIUM	LARGE
chickpeas	¼ cup ~ 50g	½ cup ~ 100g	1 cup ~ 200g
rice	¼ cup ~ 50g	⅓ cup ~ 70g	½ cup ~ 100g
lemon	⅓	½	1
tahini	½ tbsp	1 tbsp	2 tbsps

LEVEL UP! Add fresh parsley and sesame seeds.

INSTRUCTIONS

1. Soak chickpeas in plenty of water overnight. The next day, rinse and drain them.

2. Place chickpeas in a cooking pot and cover with plenty of fresh water. Bring water to a boil then lower heat to low. Cover the pot with a lid and simmer chickpeas for 30 minutes. They are cooked when tender. Drain. Alternatively, use canned chickpeas: 1 can of cooked chickpeas ~ 1 cup dry.

3. Rinse rice really well.

4. Transfer the rice to a cooking pot. Cover with double the amount of water, season for taste and stir once. Bring water to a boil then lower heat to low. Cover with a lid and simmer until it has completely absorbed the water. It will take ~ 20 minutes for white rice; 35 minutes for brown rice.

5. Add chickpeas and rice to a plate, season for taste and mix.

6. Squeeze lemon into a cup and discard it. Add tahini to the lemon juice and mix well until smooth and creamy. Drizzle it over the chickpeas with rice then garnish with fresh parsley, lemon slices and sesame seeds.

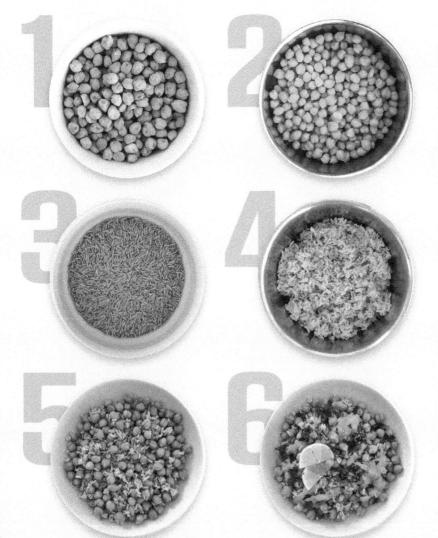

Lentil Loaf

Visual Recipe by DAREBEE
© darebee.com

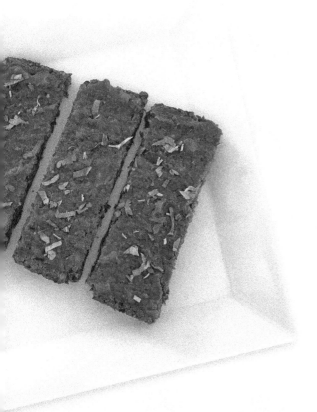

	SMALL	MEDIUM	LARGE
lentils	½ cup ~ 100g	1 cup ~ 200g	1 ½ cup ~ 300g
oat flakes	⅓ cup ~ 20g	½ cup ~ 30g	1 cup ~ 50g
tomato sauce	¼ cup ~ 50ml	⅓ cup ~ 70ml	½ cup ~ 100ml

LEVEL UP! Add fresh parsley.

INSTRUCTIONS

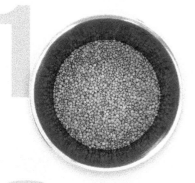
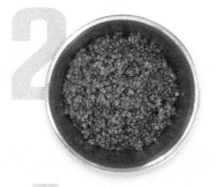
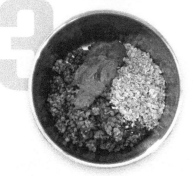
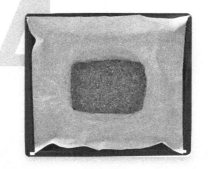
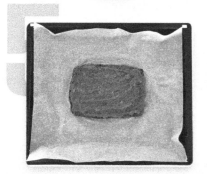
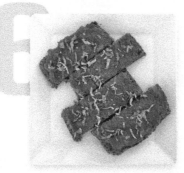

1. Rinse the lentils really well.

2. Transfer the lentils to a cooking pot. Cover with double the amount of water and stir once. Bring water to a boil then lower heat to low. Cover with a lid and simmer until the lentils are tender and have completely absorbed the water ~ 30 minutes.

3. Combine cooked lentils with oat flakes and tomato sauce, season for taste and mix well. Reserve some of the sauce for topping. Tip: use store-bought tomato sauce with basil or mushrooms in it as a shortcut.

4. Preheat the oven to 400°F (200°C). Place the lentil mix on top of a baking tray lined with baking paper and shape into a thick rectangle with a spoon. Bake in the oven for 20 minutes or until it begins to brown.

5. Take out of the oven, top with the rest of the tomato sauce and bake for another 2 minutes.

6. Transfer to a plate, cut into pieces and garnish with fresh parsley.

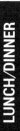

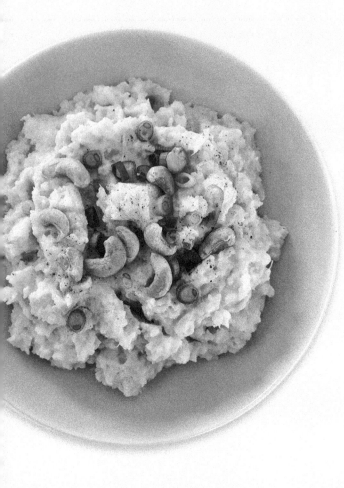

Mashed Cauliflower

Visual Recipe
by DAREBEE
© darebee.com

	SMALL	MEDIUM	LARGE
cauliflower	¼ ~ 1 cup	⅓ ~ 1 ½ cup	½ ~ 2 cups
cooking cream	1 tbsp	2 tbsps	3 tbsps

LEVEL UP! Add cashews, spring onions and black pepper.

INSTRUCTIONS

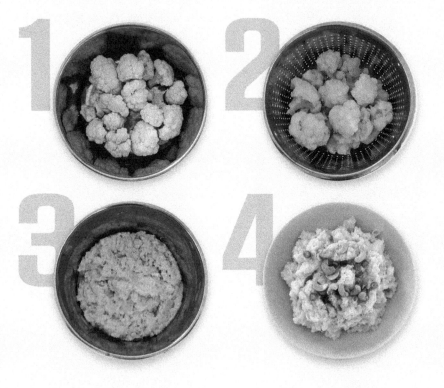

1. Separate cauliflower into florets with your hands or using a knife and wash them well.

2. Add the florets to a cooking pot and cover with water. Cover the pot with a lid, bring water to a boil then lower heat to low. Simmer for 15 minutes or until the cauliflower florets are tender. Drain.

3. Combine cauliflower with cooking cream, season for taste, and mash with a fork - or a hand blender if you like it less chunky.

4. Transfer to a plate and garnish with spring onions and top with cashews.

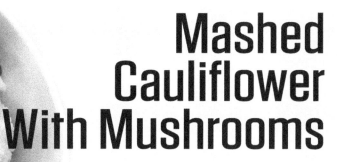

Mashed Cauliflower With Mushrooms

Visual Recipe by DAREBEE
© darebee.com

	SMALL	MEDIUM	LARGE
cauliflower	¼ ~ 1 cup	⅓ ~ 1 ½ cup	½ ~ 2 cups
cooking cream	1 tbsp	2 tbsps	3 tbsps
mushrooms	2oz ~ 60g	5oz ~ 150g	7oz ~ 200g
bell peppers	1	1	1
onion	1	1	1

LEVEL UP! Add ginger powder, garlic powder, soy sauce and sesame seeds.

INSTRUCTIONS

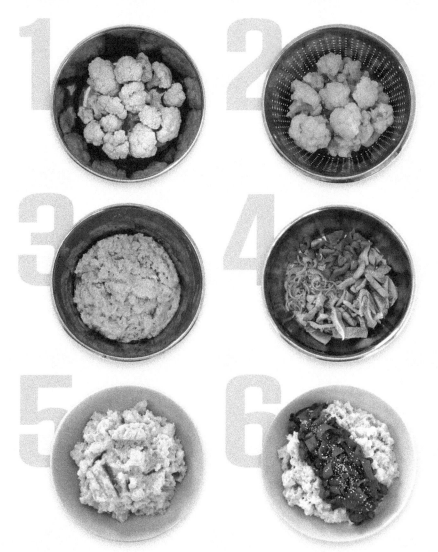

1. Separate cauliflower into florets with your hands or using a knife and wash them well.

2. Add the florets to a cooking pot and cover with water. Cover the pot with a lid, bring water to a boil then lower heat to low. Simmer for 15 minutes or until the cauliflower florets are tender. Drain.

3. Combine cauliflower with cooking cream, season for taste, and mash with a fork - or a hand blender if you like it less chunky.

4. Cut mushrooms and onion into strips and bell pepper into bite-sized pieces. Add to a frying pan and cover with ½ cup of water. Add 1 tablespoon of each - ginger powder, garlic powder and soy sauce and lemon juice, if using. Season for taste. Bring to a boil then reduce heat to medium and saute until all the water has evaporated and the mushrooms begin to become golden brown and crisp up.

5. Transfer mashed cauliflower to a plate.

6. Top with mushrooms and peppers and sprinkle with sesame seeds.

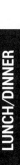

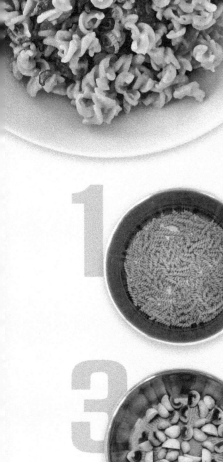

Pasta With Cream Mushrooms

Visual Recipe by DAREBEE
© darebee.com

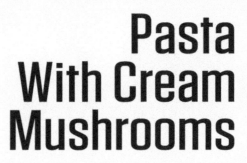

	SMALL	MEDIUM	LARGE
pasta	½ cup ~ 120g	1 ½ cup ~ 180g	2 cups ~ 180g
mushrooms	7oz ~ 200g	10oz ~ 300g	13oz ~ 400g
milk	3oz ~ 100ml	5oz ~ 150ml	7oz ~ 200ml
flour	½ tbsp	1 tbsp	1 ½ tbsp

LEVEL UP! Add spring onions.

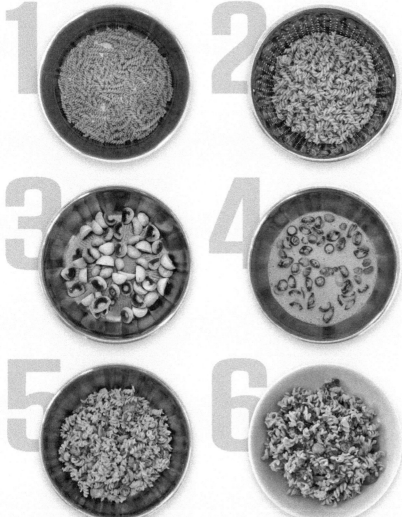

INSTRUCTIONS

1. Fill a large cooking pot with water and bring it to a boil. Add pasta and lower heat to medium.

2. Season for taste and boil the pasta for the amount of cooking time given in its packaging instructions. Alternatively, boil it until it becomes soft and no longer crunchy. Drain.

3. Add cleaned and cut mushrooms to a pot. Add 1 cup of water, season for taste and bring to a boil. Reduce heat, cover with a lid and simmer for 20 minutes or until the water evaporates.

4. Mix milk with flour and add to the mushrooms. Simmer and stir for 2 minutes or until the cream thickens.

5. Add cooked and drained pasta to mushrooms. Stir for a minute to combine.

6. Transfer to a plate and garnish with spring onions.

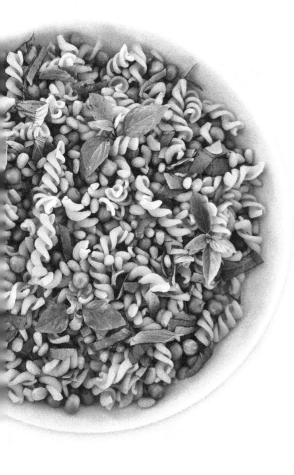

Pasta With Peas

Visual Recipe
by DAREBEE
© darebee.com

	SMALL	MEDIUM	LARGE
pasta	½ cup ~ 120g	1 ½ cup ~ 180g	2 cups ~ 180g
peas	½ cup ~ 80g	1 cup ~ 160g	1 ½ cup ~ 240g

LEVEL UP! Add fresh basil and pine nuts.

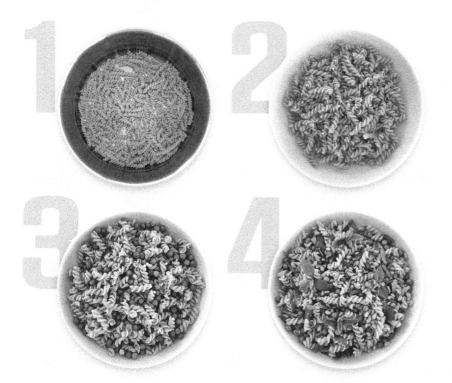

INSTRUCTIONS

1. Fill a large cooking pot with water and bring it to a boil. Add pasta and lower heat to medium. Season for taste and boil the pasta for the amount of cooking time given in its packaging instructions. Alternatively, boil it until it becomes soft and no longer crunchy.

2. Drain it and transfer to a plate.

3. Add defrosted peas.

4. Garnish with fresh basil and pine nuts.

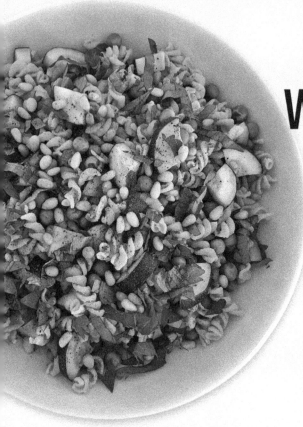

Pasta With Zucchini & Peas

Visual Recipe
by DAREBEE
© darebee.com

	SMALL	MEDIUM	LARGE
pasta	½ cup ~ 120g	1 ½ cup ~ 180g	2 cups ~ 180g
peas	½ cup ~ 80g	1 cup ~ 160g	1 ½ cup ~ 240g
zucchini	1	1	2

LEVEL UP! Add fresh parsley and pine nuts.

INSTRUCTIONS

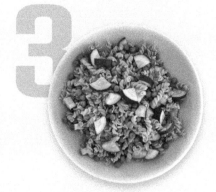
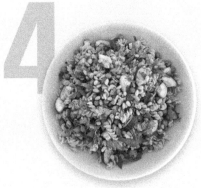
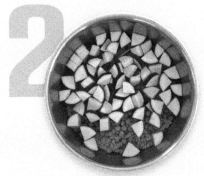
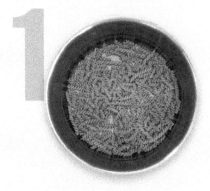

1. Fill a large cooking pot with water and bring it to a boil. Add pasta and lower heat to medium. Season for taste and boil the pasta for the amount of cooking time given in its packaging instructions. Alternatively, boil it until it becomes soft and no longer crunchy.

2. Defrost the peas and cut zucchini. Add to the boiling pasta 3 minutes before its cooking time is up.

3. Drain pasta with zucchini and peas and transfer to a plate.

4. Top it with pine nuts and garnish with parsley.

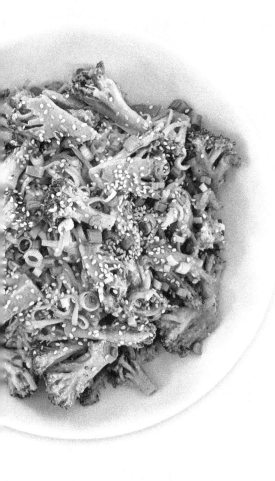

Peanut Noodles

Visual Recipe
by DAREBEE
© darebee.com

	SMALL	MEDIUM	LARGE
noodles	3oz ~ 80g	4oz ~ 120g	5oz ~ 160g
broccoli	1 cup ~ 150g	1 ½ cups ~ 220g	2 cups ~ 300g
peanut butter	1 tbsps	1 ½ tbsps	2 tbsps
soy sauce	½ tbsp	1 tbsp	1 ½ tbsp
water	2 tbsps	3 tbsp	4 tbsps

LEVEL UP! Add spring onions and sesame seeds. Add ½ tablespoon black pepper and ½ tablespoon cayenne pepper to the sauce for the extra kick.

INSTRUCTIONS

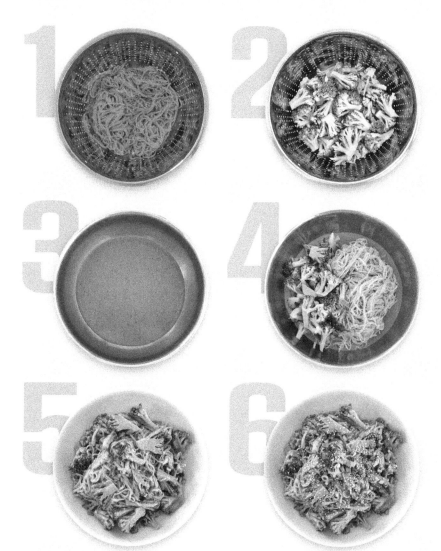

1. Fill a large cooking pot with water and bring it to a boil. Add noodles and lower heat to medium. Boil the noodles for the amount of cooking time given in its packaging instructions. Usually ~ 4 minutes. Run under cold water and drain.

2. Fill a pot with water and bring it to a boil. Add broccoli and boil it for 5 minutes or until it turns bright green. Run under cold water and drain.

3. Combine peanut butter, soy sauce and 1 cup of water together in a large frying pan. Season for taste and simmer over medium heat and stir until the sauce thickens.

4. Add broccoli and cooked noodles to the sauce. Cook and stir for another 2 minutes.

5. Transfer to a plate.

6. Garnish with spring onions and sprinkle with sesame seeds.

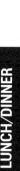

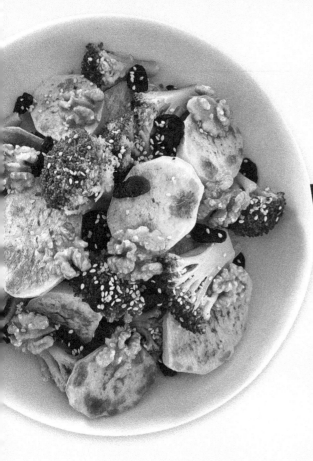

Potatoes With Broccoli

Visual Recipe by DAREBEE
Ⓒ darebee.com

	SMALL	MEDIUM	LARGE
potatoes	1 medium	2 medium	3 medium
broccoli	1 cup ~ 150g	1 ½ cups ~ 220g	2 cups ~ 300g

LEVEL UP! Add cranberries, walnuts, balsamic vinegar and sesame seeds.

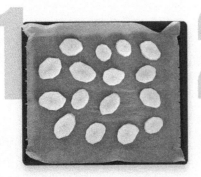
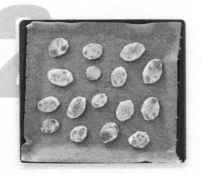
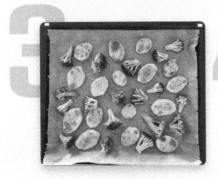
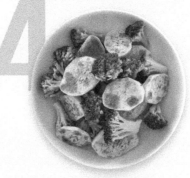
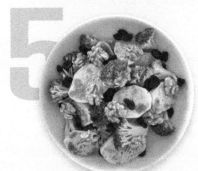
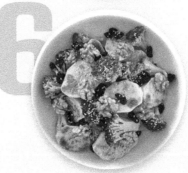

INSTRUCTIONS

1. Peel and slice the potatoes. Arrange them on top of a baking tray lined with baking paper.

2. Preheat the oven to 400ºF (200ºC). Roast the potatoes for 30 minutes or until tender. Take out of the oven and turn over.

3. Add broccoli florets and season for taste. Place back into the oven and roast for another 10 minutes. Frozen broccoli can be used and it can be taken directly from the freezer.

4. Transfer potatoes and broccoli to a plate.

5. Add dried cranberries and walnuts.

6. Drizzle with balsamic vinegar and sprinkle with sesame seeds.

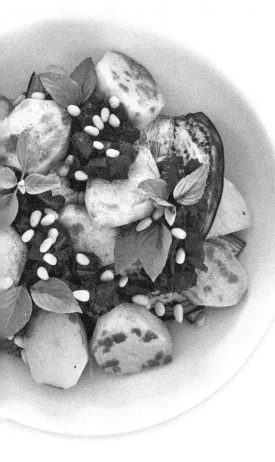

Potatoes With Eggplant

Visual Recipe
by DAREBEE
© darebee.com

	SMALL	MEDIUM	LARGE
potatoes	1	2	3
eggplant	1	2	3
tomato	1	2	3
molasses	1 tsp	2 tsps	3 tsps

LEVEL UP! Add pine nuts and fresh basil.

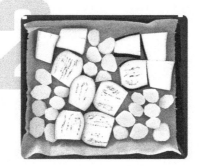

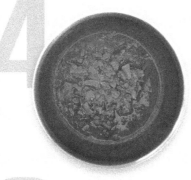

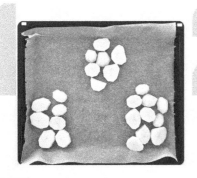

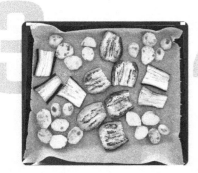

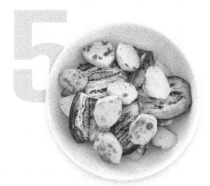

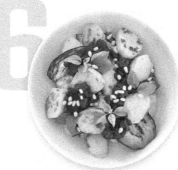

INSTRUCTIONS

1. Peel and slice the potatoes. Arrange them on top of a baking tray lined with baking paper. Preheat the oven to 400ºF (200ºC). Roast the potatoes for 20 minutes or until tender.

2. Add sliced eggplant and season for taste. Place back into the oven and roast for another 10 minutes.

3. Turn over and roast for another 10 minutes.

4. Combine diced tomato with molasses and 1 cup of water in a saucepan. Bring to a boil then lower the heat and simmer for 30 minutes or until the sauce is reduced to ⊠.

5. Transfer potatoes and eggplant to a plate.

6. Top with tomato sauce, fresh basil and pine nuts.

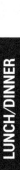

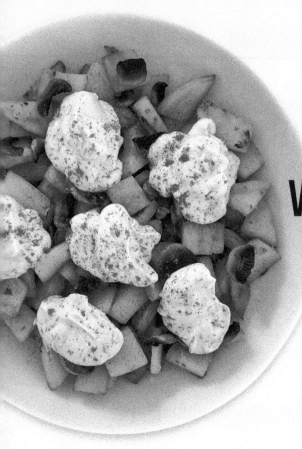

Potatoes With Mushrooms

Visual Recipe by DAREBEE
© darebee.com

	SMALL	MEDIUM	LARGE
potatoes	1 medium	2 medium	3 medium
mushrooms	7oz ~ 200g	10oz ~ 300g	13oz ~ 400g

LEVEL UP! Add plain yogurt, dried dill and cayenne pepper.

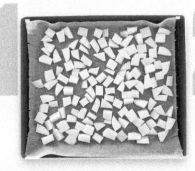
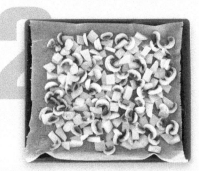
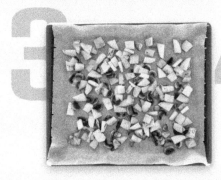
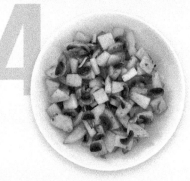
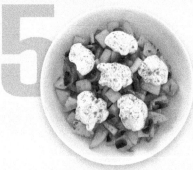

INSTRUCTIONS

1. Peel and dice the potatoes. Arrange them on top of a baking tray lined with baking paper in a single layer. Preheat the oven to 400°F (200°C). Roast in the oven for 20 minutes or until tender.

2. Add peeled and sliced mushrooms. Place back into the oven and roast for another 10 minutes.

3. Take out of the oven again. Season for taste, toss together and roast for 10 more minutes or until the potatoes and mushrooms turn golden brown.

4. Transfer the cooked potatoes and mushrooms to a plate.

5. Top with yogurt mixed with dried dill and sprinkle with cayenne pepper.

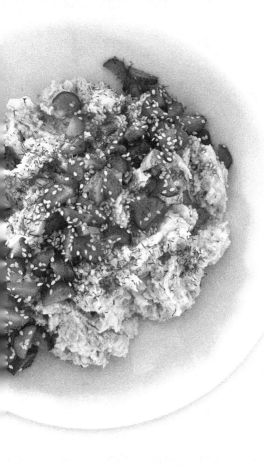

Mashed Potatoes With Pickles

Visual Recipe by DAREBEE
© darebee.com

	SMALL	MEDIUM	LARGE
potatoes	1 medium	2 medium	3 medium
tahini	1 tbsp	1 ½ tbp	2 tbsps
pickles	2	3	4

LEVEL UP! Add dried dill and sesame seeds.

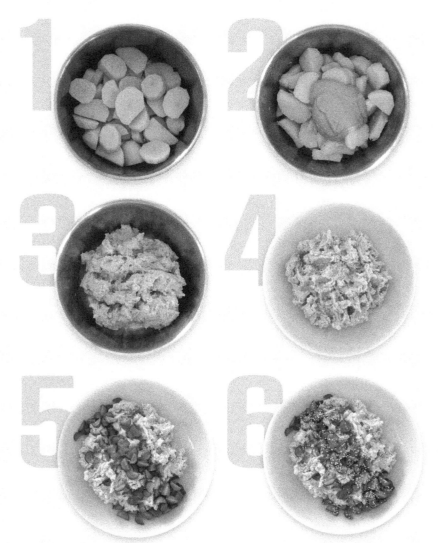

INSTRUCTIONS

1. Peel and cut the potatoes. Transfer to a cooking pot and cover with plenty of water. Bring water to a boil then lower heat to low. Cover the pot with a lid and set the timer for 30 minutes. They are cooked when tender.

2. Drain the potatoes, add tahini and a dash of water. Season for taste.

3. Mash with a fork or using a hand blender.

4. Transfer mashed potatoes to a plate.

5. Add diced pickles.

6. Sprinkle with sesame seeds and dill.

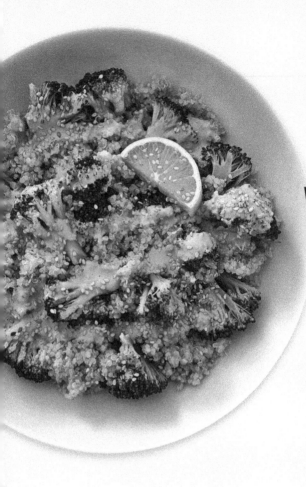

Quinoa With Broccoli

Visual Recipe
by DAREBEE
© darebee.com

	SMALL	MEDIUM	LARGE
quinoa	⅓ cup ~ 70g	½ cup ~ 100g	1 cup ~ 200g
broccoli	1 cup ~ 150g	2 cups ~ 300g	2 cups ~ 300g
tahini	1 tbsp	1 ½ tbsp	2 tbsps

LEVEL UP! Add sesame seeds and fresh lemon.

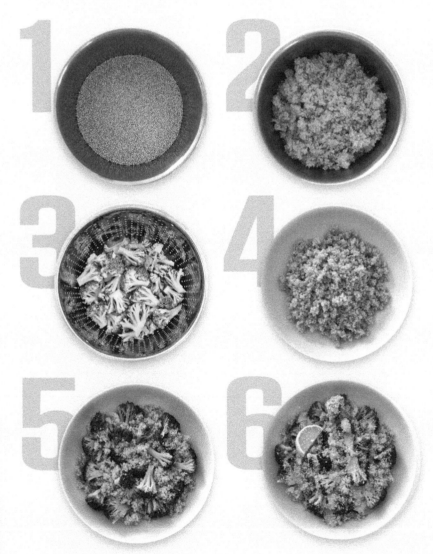

INSTRUCTIONS

1. Rinse quinoa really well.

2. Transfer the quinoa to a cooking pot. Cover with double the amount of water and stir once. Bring water to a boil then lower heat to low. Cover with a lid. Cook the quinoa until it is tender and it has completely absorbed the water ~ 15 minutes.

3. Fill a pot with water and bring it to a boil. Add broccoli and boil it for 5 minutes or until it turns bright green. Run under cold water and drain.

4. Transfer cooked quinoa to a plate.

5. Add broccoli and season for taste.

6. Drizzle with tahini thinned with water 1:3. Squeeze lemon juice on top and sprinkle with sesame seeds.

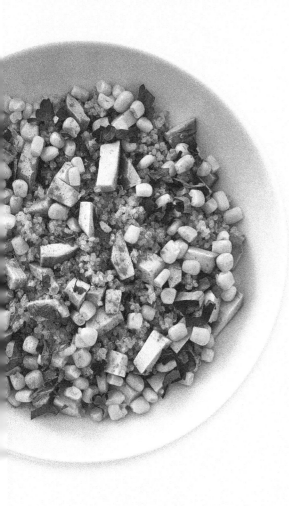

Quinoa With Corn & Avocado

Visual Recipe by DAREBEE
© darebee.com

	SMALL	MEDIUM	LARGE
quinoa	⅓ cup ~ 70g	½ cup ~ 100g	1 cup ~ 200g
corn	¼ cup ~ 40g	¼ cup ~ 40g	½ cup ~ 80g
avocado	¼	⅓	½

LEVEL UP! Add fresh parsley and cayenne pepper.

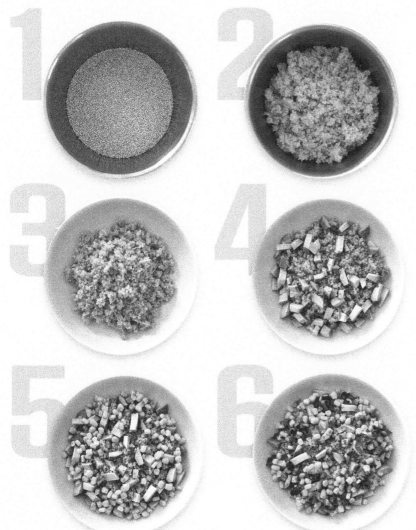

INSTRUCTIONS

1. Rinse quinoa really well.

2. Transfer the quinoa to a cooking pot. Cover with double the amount of water and stir once. Bring water to a boil then lower heat to low. Cover with a lid. Cook the quinoa until it is tender and it has completely absorbed the water ~ 15 minutes.

3. Transfer cooked quinoa to a plate.

4. Add peeled, de-stoned and diced avocado.

5. Add sweet corn and season for taste. If using frozen sweet corn, place it in a saucepan, cover with water and bring to a boil. Drain.

6. Top with fresh parsley and sprinkle with cayenne pepper.

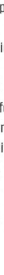

LUNCH/DINNER

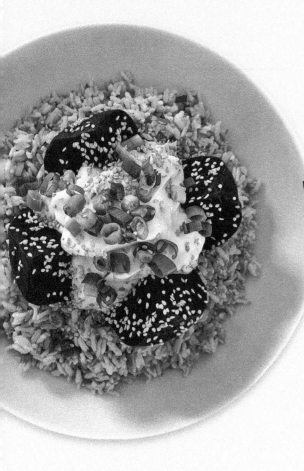

Rice
With Beetroot

Visual Recipe
by DAREBEE
© darebee.com

	SMALL	MEDIUM	LARGE
rice	⅓ cup ~ 70g	½ cup ~ 100g	1 cup ~ 200g
beetroot	1 ~ 200g	1 ~ 200g	2 ~ 400g
plain yogurt	2oz ~ 60ml	4oz ~ 120ml	6oz ~ 180ml

LEVEL UP! Add spring onions and sesame seeds.

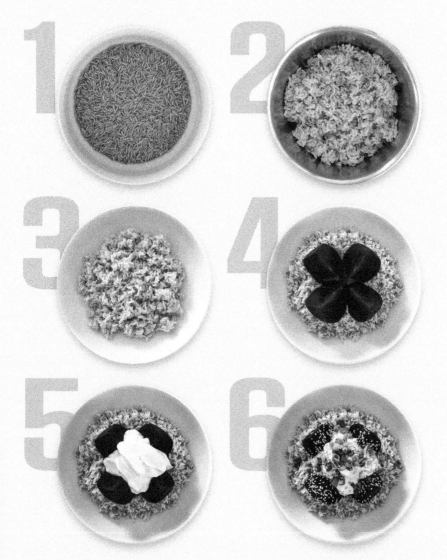

INSTRUCTIONS

1. Rinse rice really well.

2. Transfer the rice to a cooking pot. Cover with double the amount of water, season for taste and stir once. Bring water to a boil then lower heat to low. Cover with a lid and simmer until it has completely absorbed the water. It will take ~ 20 minutes for white rice; 35 minutes for brown rice.

3. Add rice to a plate.

4. Cut cooked beetroot into four, as illustrated, and nest in the middle of the rice. Season for taste.

5. Top with plain yogurt.

6. Garnish with spring onions and sesame seeds.

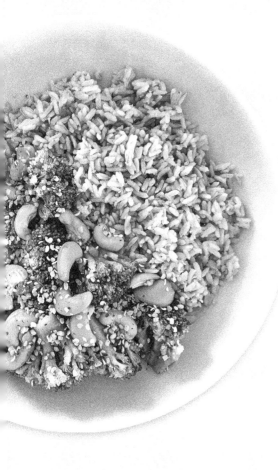

Rice With Broccoli & Cashews

Visual Recipe by DAREBEE
© darebee.com

	SMALL	MEDIUM	LARGE
rice	⅓ cup ~ 70g	½ cup ~ 100g	1 cup ~ 200g
broccoli	1 cup ~ 150g	2 cups ~ 300g	2 cups ~ 300g
cashews	5	7	10
soy sauce	1 tbsp	1 tbsp	1 tbsp
sugar	1 tsp	1 tsp	1 tsp

LEVEL UP! Add garlic powder and sesame seeds.

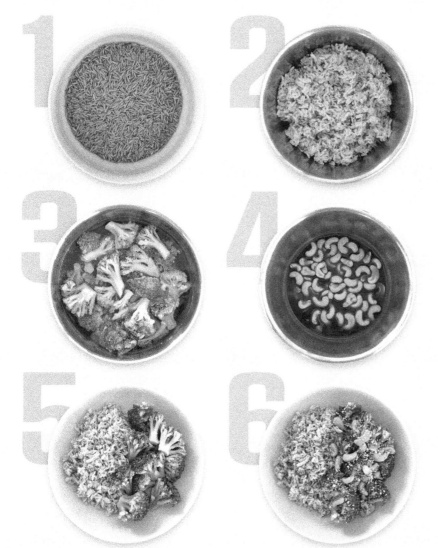

INSTRUCTIONS

1. Rinse rice really well.

2. Transfer the rice to a cooking pot. Cover with double the amount of water, season for taste and stir once. Bring water to a boil then lower heat to low. Cover with a lid and simmer until it has completely absorbed the water. It will take ~ 20 minutes for white rice; 35 minutes for brown rice.

3. Fill a pot with water and bring it to a boil. Add broccoli and boil it for 5 minutes or until it turns bright green. Run under cold water and drain.

4. Combine 1 cup of water, 1 tablespoon of soy sauce, honey or sugar, garlic powder and cashews in a saucepan. Simmer for 2 minutes and set aside.

5. Add rice and drained broccoli to a plate.

6. Pour soy sauce and cashews over the rice and broccoli and sprinkle with sesame seeds.

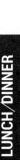

LUNCH/DINNER

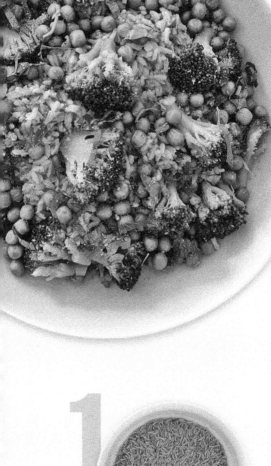

Rice With Broccoli & Peas

Visual Recipe by DAREBEE
© darebee.com

	SMALL	MEDIUM	LARGE
rice	⅓ cup ~ 70g	½ cup ~ 100g	1 cup ~ 200g
broccoli	1 cup ~ 150g	2 cups ~ 300g	2 cups ~ 300g
peas	½ cup ~ 80g	1 cup ~ 160g	1 ½ cup ~ 240g

LEVEL UP! Add fresh parsley and mustard powder.

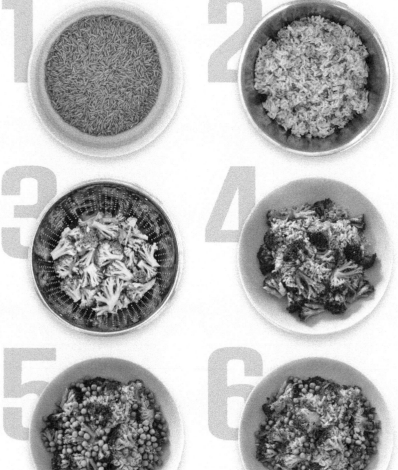

INSTRUCTIONS

1. Rinse rice really well.

2. Transfer the rice to a cooking pot. Cover with double the amount of water, season for taste and stir once. Bring water to a boil then lower heat to low. Cover with a lid and simmer until it has completely absorbed the water. It will take ~ 20 minutes for white rice; 35 minutes for brown rice.

3. Fill a pot with water and bring it to a boil. Add broccoli and boil it for 5 minutes or until it turns bright green. Run under cold water and drain.

4. Add cooked rice and cooked broccoli to a plate.

5. Add defrosted peas and season for taste.

6. Garnish with fresh parsley and sesame seeds.

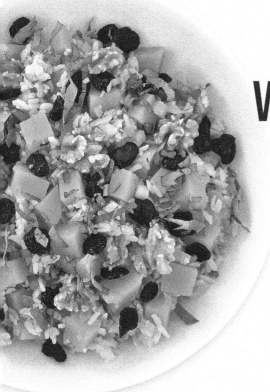

Rice With Butternut Squash

Visual Recipe by DAREBEE
© darebee.com

	SMALL	MEDIUM	LARGE
rice	⅓ cup ~ 70g	½ cup ~ 100g	1 cup ~ 200g
butternut squash	7oz ~ 200g	10oz ~ 300g	13oz ~ 400g
onion	1	1	1

LEVEL UP! Add dried cranberries, walnuts and fresh parsley and black pepper.

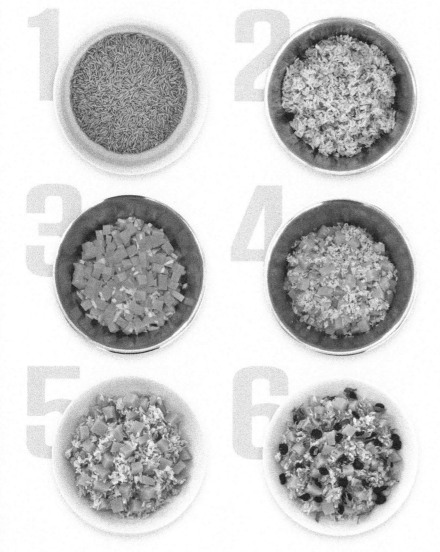

INSTRUCTIONS

1. Rinse rice really well.

2. Transfer the rice to a cooking pot. Cover with double the amount of water, season for taste and stir once. Bring water to a boil then lower heat to low. Cover with a lid and simmer until it has completely absorbed the water. It will take ~ 20 minutes for white rice; 35 minutes for brown rice.

3. Add peeled and diced butternut squash and onion to a cooking pot. Add ½ cup water and bring to a boil. Saute for 10 minutes or until butternut squash becomes soft all the way through and all the water has evaporated.

4. Add cooked rice, season for taste and mix. Cook for another 2 minutes stirring occasionally.

5. Transfer rise and butternut squash to a plate.

6. Garnish with dried cranberries, walnuts and fresh parsley.

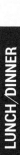

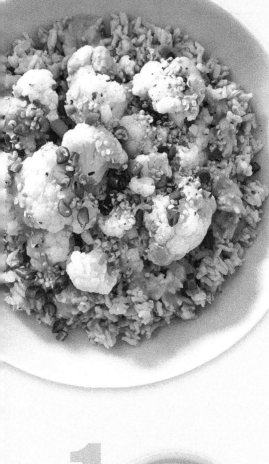

Rice With Cauliflower

Visual Recipe by DAREBEE
© darebee.com

	SMALL	MEDIUM	LARGE
rice	⅓ cup ~ 70g	½ cup ~ 100g	1 cup ~ 200g
cauliflower	¼ ~ 1 cup	⅓ ~ 1 ½ cup	½ ~ 2 cups
tahini	1 tbsp	1 ½ tbsp	2 tbsps

LEVEL UP! Add spring onions and hemp hearts.

INSTRUCTIONS

1. Rinse rice really well.

2. Transfer the rice to a cooking pot. Cover with double the amount of water, season for taste and stir once. Bring water to a boil then lower heat to low. Cover with a lid and simmer until it has completely absorbed the water. It will take ~ 20 minutes for white rice; 35 minutes for brown rice.

3. Separate cauliflower into bite-sized florets with your hands or using a knife and wash them well. Add the florets to a cooking pot and cover with water. Bring water to a boil then lower heat to low. Simmer for 15 minutes or until the cauliflower florets are soft all the way through. Drain.

4. Add cooked rice to a plate.

5. Add cooked cauliflower to the rice and season for taste.

6. Drizzle with tahini thinned with water 1:3. Top with spring onions and hemp hearts.

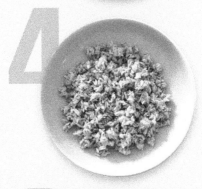
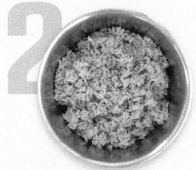
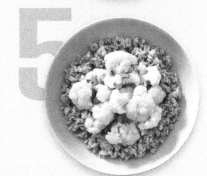
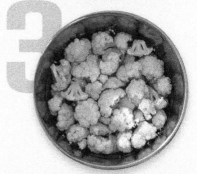
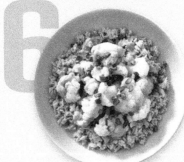
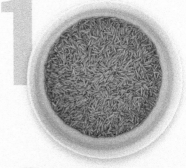

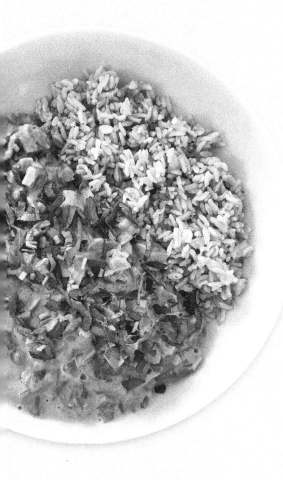

Rice With Cream Mushrooms

Visual Recipe
by DAREBEE
© darebee.com

	SMALL	MEDIUM	LARGE
rice	⅓ cup ~ 70g	½ cup ~ 100g	1 cup ~ 200g
mushrooms	7oz ~ 200g	10oz ~ 300g	13oz ~ 400g
onion	1	1	1
milk	3oz ~ 100ml	5oz ~ 150ml	7oz ~ 200ml
flour	½ tbsp	1 tbsp	1 ½ tbsp

LEVEL UP! Add fresh parsley and black pepper.

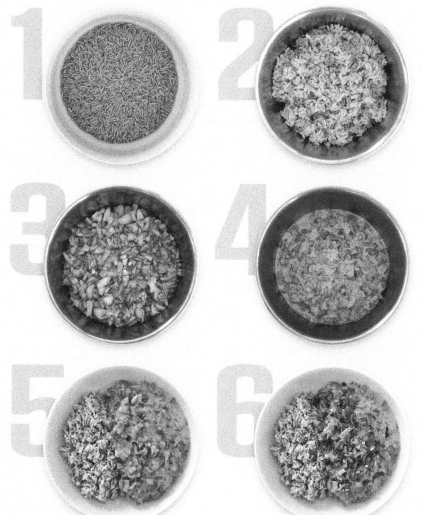

INSTRUCTIONS

1. Rinse rice really well.

2. Transfer the rice to a cooking pot. Cover with double the amount of water, season for taste and stir once. Bring water to a boil then lower heat to low. Cover with a lid and simmer until it has completely absorbed the water. It will take ~ 20 minutes for white rice; 35 minutes for brown rice.

3. Add diced mushrooms and onion to a pot. Add 1 cup of water and bring to a boil. Reduce heat, cover with a lid and simmer for 20 minutes or until the water evaporates.

4. Mix milk with flour and add to the mushrooms. Season for taste, simmer and stir for 2 minutes or until the cream thickens.

5. Add rice and cream mushrooms to a plate.

6. Top with fresh parsley and sprinkle with black pepper.

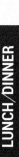

LUNCH/DINNER

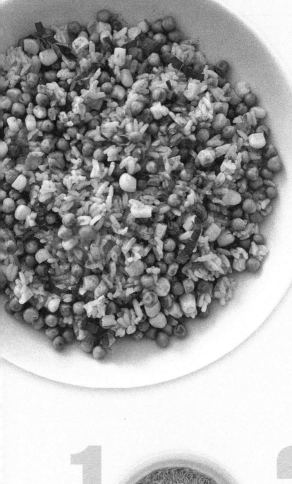

Rice With Peas & Corn

Visual Recipe
by DAREBEE
© darebee.com

	SMALL	MEDIUM	LARGE
rice	⅓ cup ~ 70g	½ cup ~ 100g	1 cup ~ 200g
peas	½ cup ~ 80g	1 cup ~ 160g	1 ½ cup ~ 240g
corn	¼ cup ~ 40g	¼ cup ~ 40g	½ cup ~ 80g

LEVEL UP! Add fresh parsley and cayenne pepper.

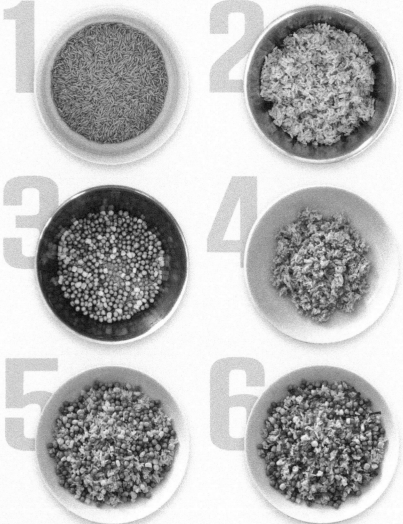

INSTRUCTIONS

1. Rinse rice really well.

2. Transfer the rice to a cooking pot. Cover with double the amount of water, season for taste and stir once. Bring water to a boil then lower heat to low. Cover with a lid and simmer until it has completely absorbed the water. It will take ~ 20 minutes for white rice; 35 minutes for brown rice.

3. Combine peas and corn, both can be taken directly from a freezer, in a saucepan. Add ½ cup of water and bring to a boil. Remove from heat, drain.

4. Add rice to a plate.

5. Add drained corn and peas. Season for taste.

6. Garnish with fresh parsley and sprinkle with cayenne pepper.

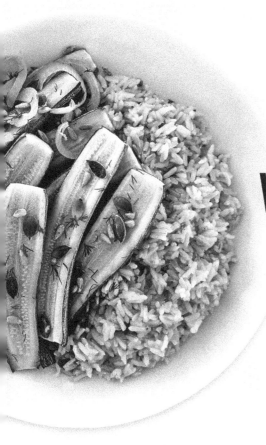

Rice
With Zucchini

Visual Recipe
by DAREBEE
© darebee.com

	SMALL	MEDIUM	LARGE
rice	⅓ cup ~ 70g	½ cup ~ 100g	1 cup ~ 200g
zucchini	1	2	3
onion	1	1	1

LEVEL UP! Add dill, pumpkin and sunflower seeds.

INSTRUCTIONS

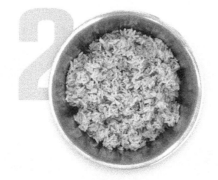

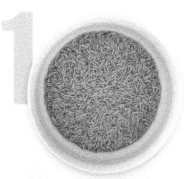

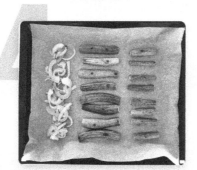

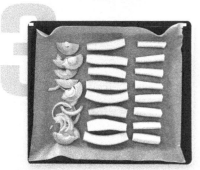

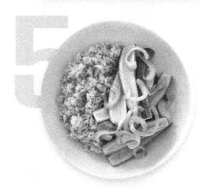

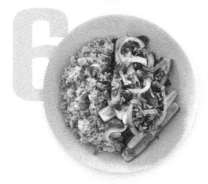

1. Rinse rice really well.

2. Transfer the rice to a cooking pot. Cover with double the amount of water, season for taste and stir once. Bring water to a boil then lower heat to low. Cover with a lid and simmer until it has completely absorbed the water. It will take ~ 20 minutes for white rice; 35 minutes for brown rice.

3. Slice zucchini and onion. Transfer to a baking tray lined with baking paper.

4. Preheat the oven to 400°F (200°C). Roast in the oven for 20 minutes.

5. Add cooked rice and roasted vegetables to a plate. Season for taste.

6. Top with dill, sunflower and pumpkin seeds.

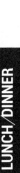

LUNCH/DINNER

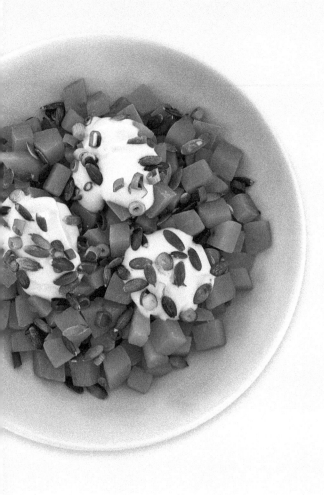

Roasted Butternut Squash With Yogurt

Visual Recipe
by DAREBEE
© darebee.com

	SMALL	MEDIUM	LARGE
butternut squash	7oz ~ 200g	10oz ~ 300g	13oz ~ 400g
plain yogurt	2oz ~ 60ml	4oz ~ 120ml	6oz ~ 180ml

LEVEL UP! Add spring onions and pumpkin seeds.

1 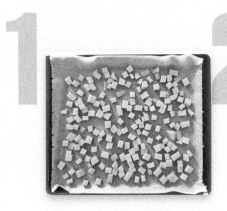 **2** 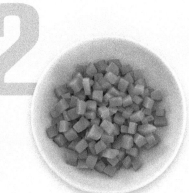 **3**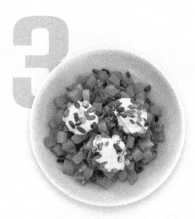

INSTRUCTIONS

1. Peel and dice butternut squash. Transfer to a baking tray lined with baking paper, arrange in a single layer and season for taste. Preheat the oven to 400°F (200°C). Roast butternut squash in the middle of the oven for 20 minutes or until it's soft all the way through.

2. Transfer to a plate.

3. Top with yogurt. Garnish with spring onions and pumpkin seeds.

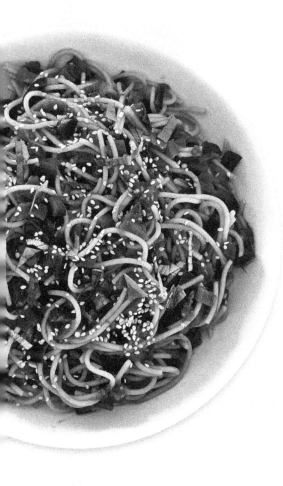

Spaghetti With Tomato & Eggplant

Visual Recipe
by DAREBEE
© darebee.com

	SMALL	MEDIUM	LARGE
spaghetti	3oz ~ 90g	6oz ~ 180g	8oz ~ 250g
tomato	1	1	2
eggplant	1	1	2
molasses	1 tsp	1 tsps	2 tsps

LEVEL UP! Add fresh basil, cinnamon and sesame seeds.

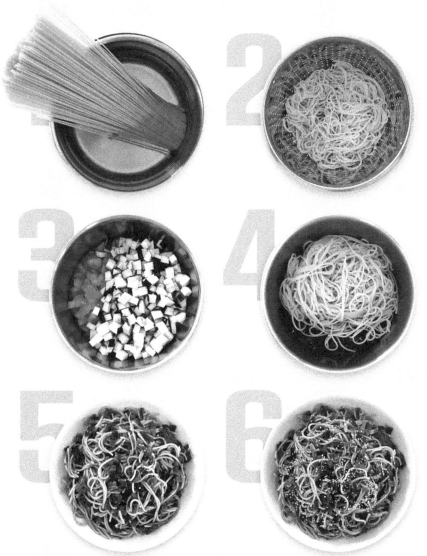

INSTRUCTIONS

1. Fill a large cooking pot with water and bring it to a boil. Add spaghetti and lower heat to medium.

2. Boil the spaghetti for the amount of cooking time given in its packaging instructions. Alternatively, boil it until it becomes soft and no longer crunchy. Drain.

3. Combine diced tomato, diced eggplant, molasses, cinnamon - if using, and 1 cup of water in a cooking pot. Season for taste. Mix well and bring to a boil. Lower heat to medium and simmer for 30 minutes or until all the water is almost gone.

4. Add cooked spaghetti to the tomato and eggplant sauce and mix well until it is fully coated.

5. Transfer to a plate.

6. Garnish with fresh basil and sprinkle with sesame seeds.

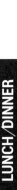

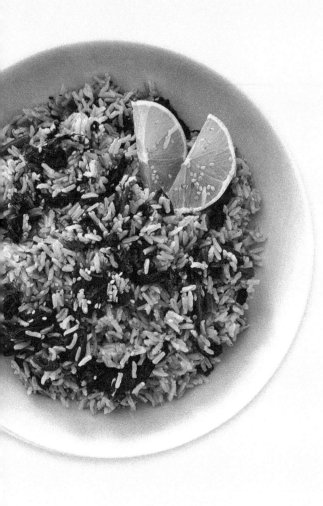

Spinach Rice

Visual Recipe by DAREBEE
© darebee.com

	SMALL	MEDIUM	LARGE
rice	⅓ cup ~ 70g	½ cup ~ 100g	1 cup ~ 200g
frozen spinach	½ cup ~ 80g	1 cup ~ 160g	1 ½ cup ~ 240g

LEVEL UP! Add lemon, sun-dried tomatoes and sesame seeds.

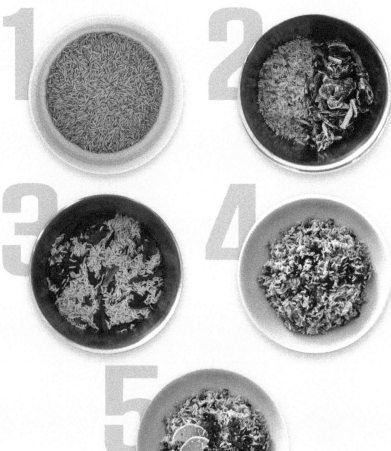

INSTRUCTIONS

1. Rinse rice really well.

2. Transfer the rice and the frozen spinach to a cooking pot. Cover with double the amount of water, season for taste and stir once.

3. Bring water to a boil then lower heat to low. Cover with a lid and simmer until it has completely absorbed the water. It will take ~ 20 minutes for white rice; 35 minutes for brown rice.

4. Transfer to a plate.

5. Add chopped up sun-dried tomatoes and drizzle with lemon juice. Add extra lemon slices for garnish and sprinkle with sesame seeds.

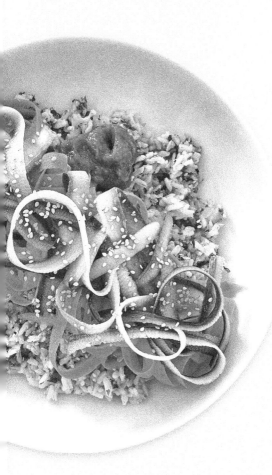

Sushi Rice

Visual Recipe
by DAREBEE
© darebee.com

	SMALL	MEDIUM	LARGE
rice	⅓ cup ~ 70g	½ cup ~ 100g	1 cup ~ 200g
seaweed flakes	1 tbsp	1 ½ tbsp	2 tbsps
carrot	1	1	1
cucumber	1	1	1
rice vinegar	1 tbsp	1 ½ tbsp	2 tbsps

LEVEL UP! Add umeboshi paste and sesame seeds.

INSTRUCTIONS

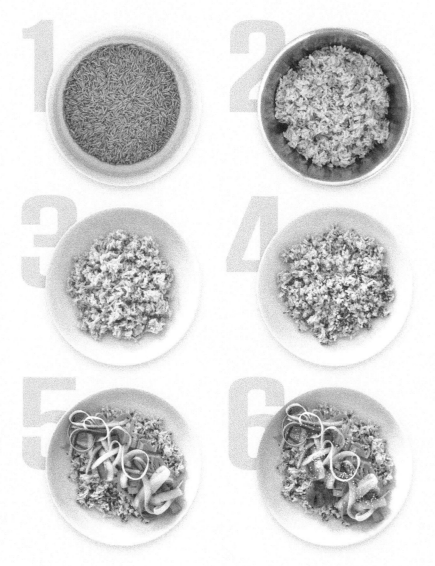

1. Rinse rice really well.

2. Transfer the rice to a cooking pot. Cover with double the amount of water, season for taste and stir once. Bring water to a boil then lower heat to low. Cover with a lid and simmer until it has completely absorbed the water. It will take ~ 20 minutes for white rice; 35 minutes for brown rice.

3. Add rice to a plate.

4. Add seaweed flakes and mix well.

5. Use a potato peeler and cut cucumber and peeled carrot into strips. Arrange on top of the rice.

6. Drizzle with rice vinegar, sprinkle with sesame seeds. If on hand, add 1 tablespoon of umeboshi paste. Tip: you can use sushi vinegar instead of rice vinegar.

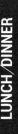

LUNCH/DINNER

Sushi Rolls

Visual Recipe
by DAREBEE
© darebee.com

	SMALL	MEDIUM	LARGE
rice	½ cup ~ 100g	⅔ cup ~ 130g	1 cup ~ 200g
rice vinegar	1 tbsp	1 ½ tbsp	2 tbsps
nori sheets	2	3	4
avocado	⅓	½	1
cucumber	1	1	1

LEVEL UP! Add sesame seeds and soy sauce.

INSTRUCTIONS

1. Rinse rice really well.

2. Transfer the rice to a cooking pot. Cover with double the amount of water, season for taste and stir once. Bring water to a boil then lower heat to low. Cover with a lid and simmer until it has completely absorbed the water. It will take ~ 20 minutes for white rice; 35 minutes for brown rice. Combine rice with vinegar (or sushi seasoning) and set aside.

3. Take some of the rice and place it all over the nori sheet leaving about ½ inch (~1cm) at the top. Flatten the rice with the flat part of the knife.

4. Quarter the cucumber lengthwise, cut out the seeds and slice it into thin strips. Cut the avocado into two lengthwise, remove the stone. Use a blunt knife to cut out slices directly from the shell as you would with butter. Place the cucumber and avocado cut into strips on top of the rice, towards the bottom.

5. Fold the mat to make a roll.

6. Cut each roll in half, then cut each half in half then cut those pieces in half. Sprinkle with sesame seeds. Serve with a side of soy sauce.

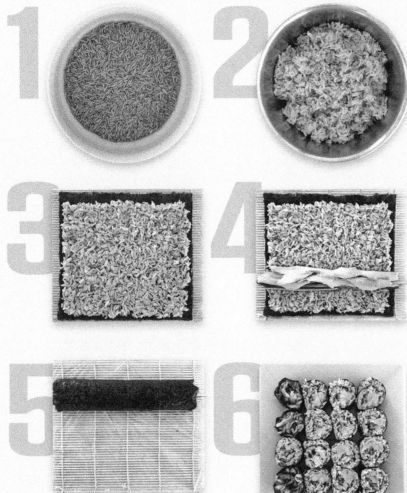

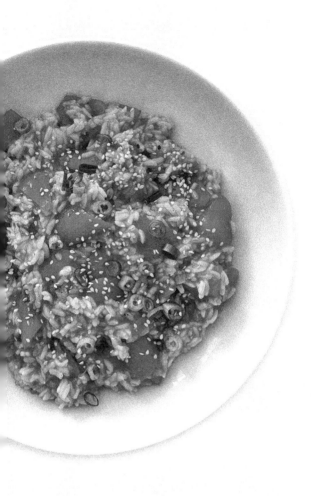

Sweet & Sour Rice

Visual Recipe
by DAREBEE
© darebee.com

	SMALL	MEDIUM	LARGE
rice	⅓ cup ~ 70g	½ cup ~ 100g	1 cup ~ 200g
bell pepper	1	2	3
rice flour	1 tbsp	1 tbsp	1 ½ tbsp
rice vinegar	¼ cup ~ 50ml	½ cup ~ 100ml	½ cup ~ 100ml
maple syrup	¼ cup ~ 60ml	⅓ cup ~ 80ml	½ cup ~ 120ml
water	½ cup ~ 100ml	⅔ cup ~ 130ml	1 cup ~ 200ml

LEVEL UP! Add spring onions and sesame seeds.

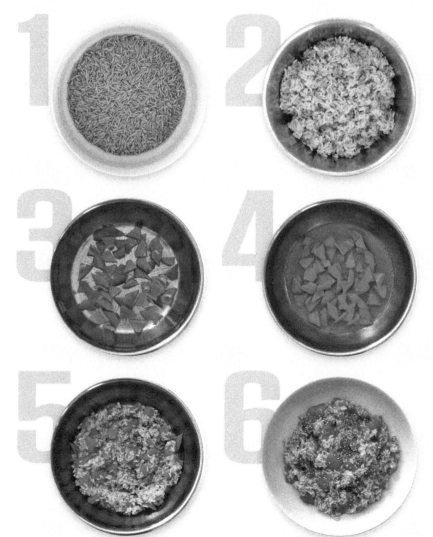

INSTRUCTIONS

1. Rinse rice really well.

2. Transfer the rice to a cooking pot. Cover with double the amount of water, season for taste and stir once. Bring water to a boil then lower heat to low. Cover with a lid and simmer until it has completely absorbed the water. It will take ~ 20 minutes for white rice; 35 minutes for brown rice.

3. Clean and cut bell peppers into bite-sized pieces and add to a large frying pan.

4. Add vinegar, maple syrup, flour and water to a mixing bowl. Stir until combined and pour over the peppers. Bring to a boil then reduce heat to medium, cook for 10 minutes stirring occasionally until the sauce thickens and the water is reduced to a third of the original amount.

5. Add the rice to the pan, cook and stir for another 2 minutes. Season for taste.

6. Transfer to a plate. Garnish with spring onions and sprinkle with sesame seeds.

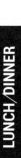

LUNCH / DINNER

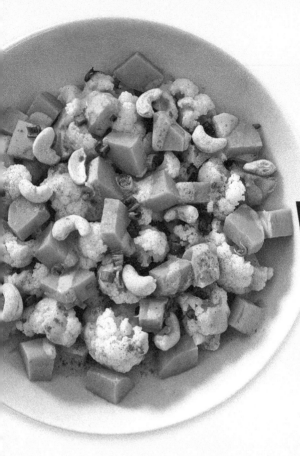

Sweet Potato With Cauliflower

Visual Recipe by DAREBEE
© darebee.com

	SMALL	MEDIUM	LARGE
sweet potato	1 small	1	2
cauliflower	¼ ~ 1 cup	⅓ ~ 1 ½ cup	½ ~ 2 cups
tahini	1 tbsp	1 ½ tbsp	2 tbsps

LEVEL UP! Add cashews, spring onion and cumin.

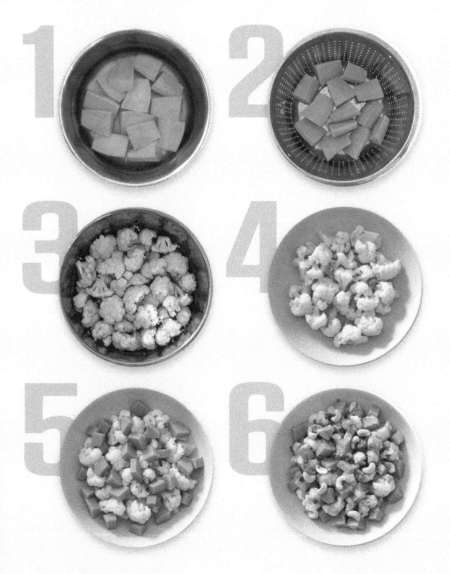

INSTRUCTIONS

1. Add peeled and cut sweet potato to a cooking pot and cover with water. Bring water to a boil then lower heat to low. Simmer for 15 minutes or until the potatoes are soft all the way through.

2. Drain the potatoes and set aside.

3. Separate cauliflower into bite-sized florets with your hands or using a knife and wash them well. Add the florets to a cooking pot and cover with water. Bring water to a boil then lower heat to low. Simmer for 15 minutes or until the cauliflower florets are soft all the way through.

4. Drain and transfer to a plate.

5. Add cooked sweet potatoes and season for taste.

6. Drizzle with tahini thinned with water 1:3. Top with cashews and spring onion and sprinkle with cumin.

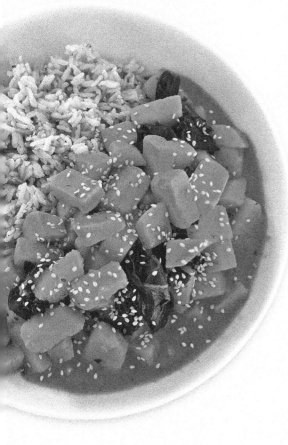

Sweet Potato Curry with Rice

Visual Recipe
by DAREBEE
© darebee.com

	SMALL	MEDIUM	LARGE
sweet potato	1 small	1	2
rice	¼ cup ~ 50g	⅓ cup ~ 70g	½ cup ~ 100g
frozen spinach	¼ cup ~ 40g	½ cup ~ 80g	1 cup ~ 160g
tomato paste	1 tbsp	2 tbsps	3 tbsps
coconut milk	3oz ~ 100ml	5oz ~ 150ml	7oz ~ 200ml
curry powder	½ tbsp	1 tbsp	1 ½ tbsp

LEVEL UP! Add sesame seeds.

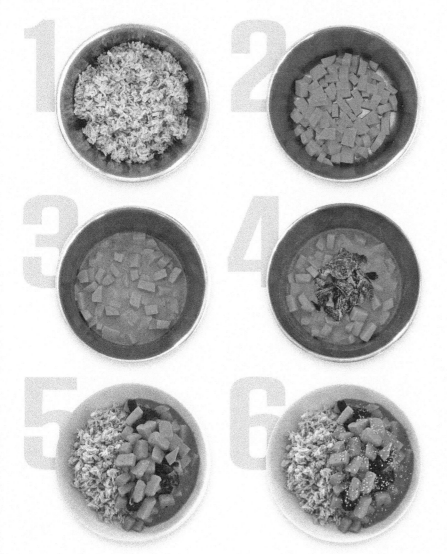

INSTRUCTIONS

1. Rinse rice really well. Transfer the rice to a cooking pot. Cover with double the amount of water, season for taste and stir once. Bring water to a boil then lower heat to low. Cover with a lid and simmer until it has completely absorbed the water. It will take ~ 20 minutes for white rice; 35 minutes for brown rice.

2. Peel and cut sweet potato into bite-sized pieces. Cover with 1 cup of water. Cover with a lid and bring to a boil. Saute for 10 minutes or until tender. Drain.

3. Combine coconut milk, curry powder and tomato paste together and pour over the potatoes.

4. Add spinach - can be taken directly from the freezer, season for taste and stir. Cook for another 2-3 minutes or until the curry thickens.

5. Add cooked rice to one side of the plate and add ready sweet potato curry to the other.

6. Sprinkle with sesame seeds.

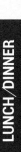

LUNCH/DINNER

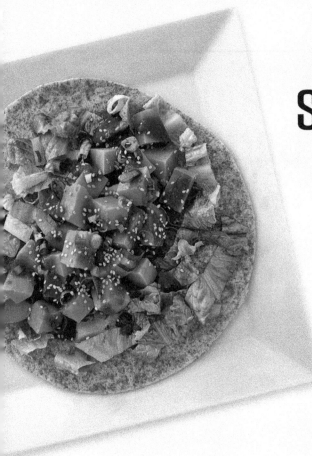

Sweet Potato Tortilla Wrap

Visual Recipe by DAREBEE
© darebee.com

	SMALL	MEDIUM	LARGE
sweet potato	1 small	1	2
tortilla wrap	1	1	2
lettuce	1 cup ~ 50g	1 cup ~ 50g	1 cup ~ 50g

LEVEL UP! Add miso paste, spring onions and sesame seeds.

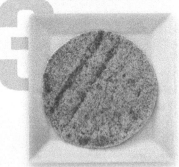
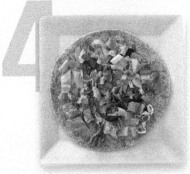
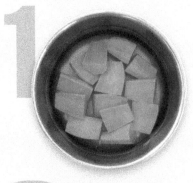
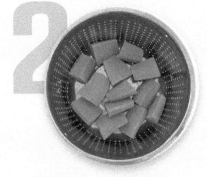
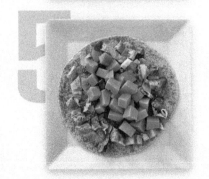
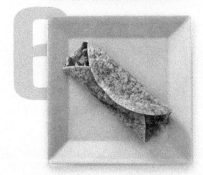

INSTRUCTIONS

1. Add peeled and cut sweet potato to a cooking pot and cover with water. Bring water to a boil then lower heat to low. Simmer for 15 minutes or until the potatoes are soft all the way through.

2. Drain the potatoes and set aside.

3. Toast tortilla in the oven for 2 minutes.

4. Add cut lettuce.

5. Add sweet potato and season for taste.

6. Thin miso paste, if using, with water 1:1 ratio and drizzle over the potatoes. Garnish with spring onions and sesame seeds. Fold it up.

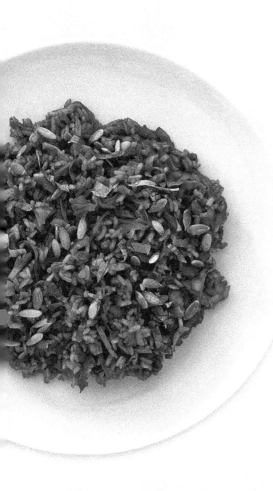

Tomato Cabbage Rice

Visual Recipe
by DAREBEE
© darebee.com

	SMALL	MEDIUM	LARGE
rice	⅓ cup ~ 70g	½ cup ~ 100g	1 cup ~ 200g
cabbage	1 cup ~ 50g	2 cups ~ 100g	3 cups ~ 150g
tomato paste	1 tbsp	2 tbsps	3 tbsps
molasses	1 tsp	2 tsps	3 tsps
water	¼ cup ~ 50ml	⅓ cup ~ 70ml	½ cup ~ 100ml

LEVEL UP! Add fresh parsley and pumpkin seeds.

INSTRUCTIONS

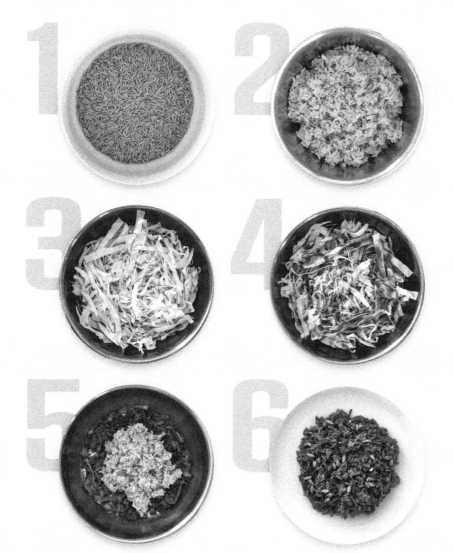

1. Rinse rice really well.

2. Transfer the rice to a cooking pot. Cover with double the amount of water, season for taste and stir once. Bring water to a boil then lower heat to low. Cover with a lid and simmer until it has completely absorbed the water. It will take ~ 20 minutes for white rice; 35 minutes for brown rice.

3. Cut cabbage into strips and transfer to a deep frying pan.

4. Mix together water, tomato paste and molasses and stir until combined. Pour over the cabbage. Bring to a boil, lower the heat to medium and simmer for 10 minutes or until all the liquid has evaporated.

5. Add rice, season for taste and toss together. Cook for another 2 minutes.

6. Transfer to a plate and garnish with fresh parsley and top with pumpkin seeds.

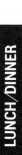

LUNCH/DINNER

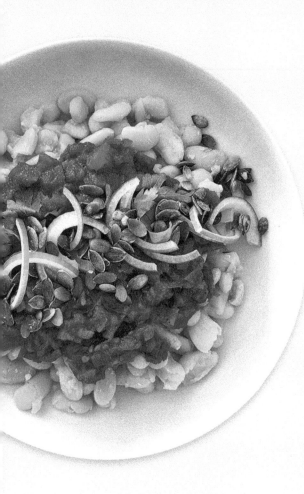

White Beans With Tomato Sauce

Visual Recipe by DAREBEE
© darebee.com

	SMALL	MEDIUM	LARGE
white beans	¼ cup ~ 50g	½ cup ~ 100g	1 cup ~ 200g
tomato	1	1	2
onion	1	1	1
molasses	1 tsp	1 tsp	2 tsps

LEVEL UP! Add fresh parsley and pumpkin seeds.

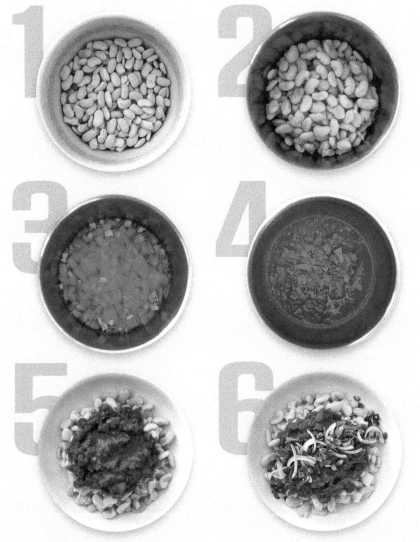

INSTRUCTIONS

1. Soak beans in plenty of water overnight. The next day, rinse and drain them.

2. Place the beans in a large cooking pot and cover with plenty of fresh water. Bring water to a boil then lower heat to low. Cover the pot with a lid. Simmer the beans until tender ~ 30 minutes. Drain. Alternatively, use canned beans: 1 can of cooked beans ~ 1 cup dry.

3. Combine diced tomato with molasses and 1 cup of water in a saucepan. Season for taste and stir.

4. Bring to a boil then lower the heat and simmer for 30 minutes or until the sauce is reduced to ⅓.

5. Drain the beans and transfer to a plate. Cover the beans with the tomato sauce.

6. Top with onion, parsley and pumpkin seeds.

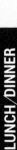

LUNCH/DINNER

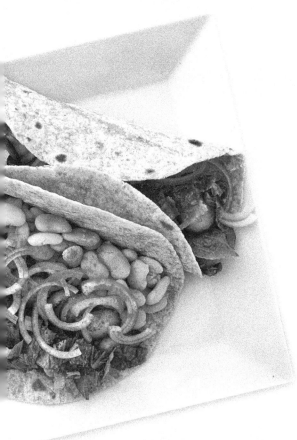

White Bean Tortilla Wrap

Visual Recipe by DAREBEE
© darebee.com

	SMALL	MEDIUM	LARGE
white beans	¼ cup ~ 50g	½ cup ~ 100g	1 cup ~ 200g
tortilla wrap	1	1	2
cucumber	1	1	1
lettuce	1 cup ~ 50g	1 cup ~ 50g	1 cup ~ 50g

LEVEL UP! Add red onion and cayenne pepper.

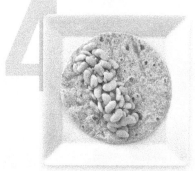
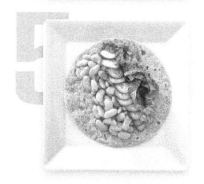
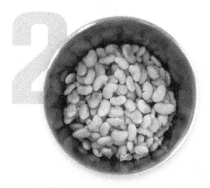
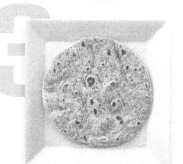
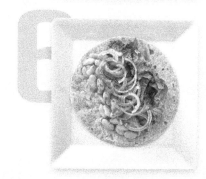
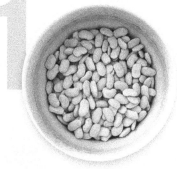

INSTRUCTIONS

1. Soak beans in plenty of water overnight. The next day, rinse and drain them.

2. Place the beans in a large cooking pot and cover with plenty of fresh water. Bring water to a boil then lower heat to low. Cover the pot with a lid. Simmer the beans until tender ~ 30 minutes. Drain. Alternatively, use canned beans: 1 can of cooked beans ~ 1 cup dry.

3. Toast tortillas in the oven for 2 minutes.

4. Fill each tortilla wrap with beans.

5. Add sliced cucumbers and lettuce and season for taste.

6. Top with sliced onions and sprinkle with cayenne pepper.

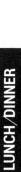

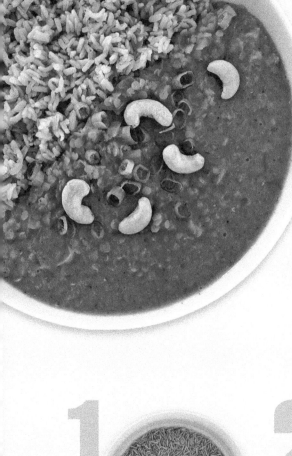

Yellow Lentil Curry with Rice

Visual Recipe by DAREBEE
© darebee.com

	SMALL	MEDIUM	LARGE
yellow lentils	¼ cup ~ 50g	½ cup ~ 100g	1 cup ~ 200g
rice	¼ cup ~ 50g	⅓ cup ~ 70g	½ cup ~ 100g
onion	1	1	1
green pepper	1	1	1
tomato	1	1	1
milk	3oz ~ 100ml	5oz ~ 150ml	7oz ~ 200ml
molasses	1 tsp	1 ½ tsp	2 tsps
curry powder	½ tbsp	1 tbsp	1 ½ tbsp

LEVEL UP! Add spring onions and cashews.

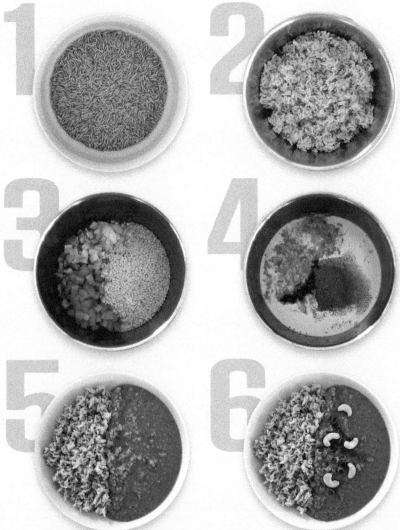

INSTRUCTIONS

1. Rinse rice really well.

2. Transfer the rice to a cooking pot. Cover with double the amount of water, season for taste and stir once. Bring water to a boil then lower heat to low. Cover with a lid and simmer until it has completely absorbed the water. It will take ~ 20 minutes for white rice; 35 minutes for brown rice.

3. Combine diced green pepper, onion and tomato in a cooking pot. Add yellow lentils and equal amount of water 1:1 ratio. Mix everything together and bring to a boil. Cook for 10 minutes until water has almost evaporated and the lentils are tender.

4. Add milk, molasses and curry powder to the lentils, season for taste and stir. Cook for another 2-3 minutes or until the curry thickens.

5. Add cooked rice to one side of the plate and ready lentil curry to the other.

6. Top with spring onions and cashew nuts.

LUNCH / DINNER

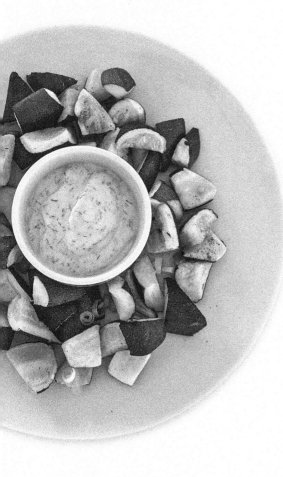

Zucchini With Yogurt Sauce

Visual Recipe by DAREBEE
© darebee.com

	SMALL	MEDIUM	LARGE
zucchini	2	3	4
plain yogurt	3oz ~ 100ml	7oz ~ 200ml	8oz ~ 240ml

LEVEL UP! Add spring onions, 1 tsp dill, 1 tsp fresh or powdered garlic and black pepper.

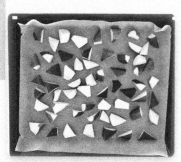
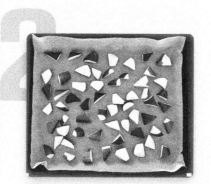
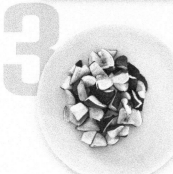
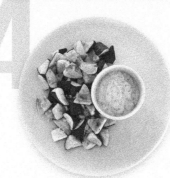

INSTRUCTIONS

1. Cut zucchini into bite-sized pieces and arrange on top of a baking tray lined with baking paper. Season for taste.

2. Preheat the oven to 400ºF (200ºC). Roast zucchini in the middle of the oven for 10 minutes or until it's soft all the way through and beginning to brown.

3. Transfer to a plate.

4. Mix plain yogurt, dried or fresh dill and garlic together to make the sauce. Season for taste and place alongside zucchini. Garnish zucchini with spring onions and sprinkle with black pepper.

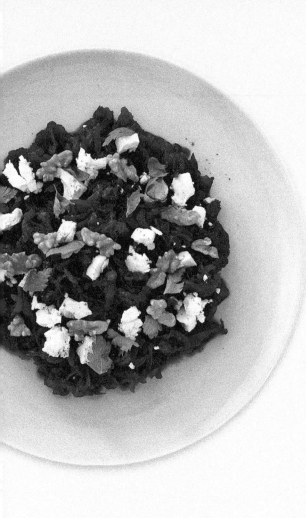

Beetroot Salad

Visual Recipe
by DAREBEE
© darebee.com

	SMALL	MEDIUM	LARGE
cooked beetroot	1	2	3
balsamic vinegar	1 tbsp	2 tbsps	3 tbsp
molasses	1 tsp	2 tsps	3 tsps

LEVEL UP! Add white cheese, fresh parsley, garlic - fresh or powdered, and walnuts.

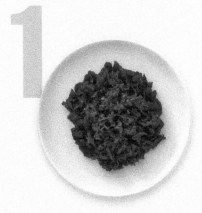  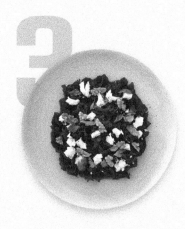

INSTRUCTIONS

1. Grate cooked beetroot and transfer to a plate.

2. Combine balsamic vinegar with molasses and garlic, if using. If using fresh garlic, crush it or finely dice it first. Stir well and season for taste. Drizzle the sauce over the beetroot. Crumble white cheese on top.

3. Garnish with fresh parsley and walnuts.

SALADS

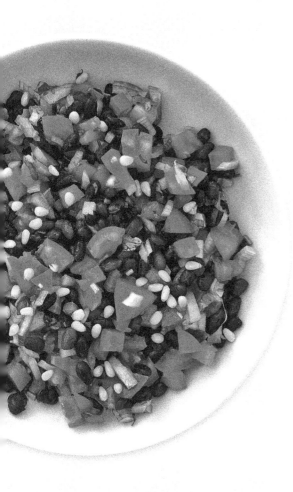

Black Bean Salad

Visual Recipe
by DAREBEE
© darebee.com

	SMALL	MEDIUM	LARGE
black beans	¼ cup ~ 50g	½ cup ~ 100g	1 cup ~ 200g
tomato	1	1	2
onion	1	1	2

LEVEL UP! Add balsamic vinegar, pine nuts and parsley.

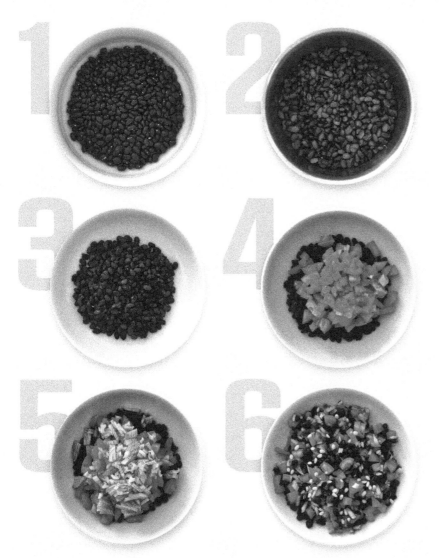

INSTRUCTIONS

1. Soak beans in plenty of water overnight. The next day, rinse and drain them.

2. Place the beans in a large cooking pot and cover with plenty of fresh water. Bring water to a boil then lower heat to low. Cover the pot with a lid. Simmer the beans until tender ~ 45-60 minutes. Drain. Alternatively, use canned beans: 1 can of cooked beans ~ 1 cup dry.

3. Drain the beans and transfer to a plate.

4. Add diced tomatoes.

5. Add diced onions, season for taste and mix well.

6. Add parsley and pine nuts and mix.

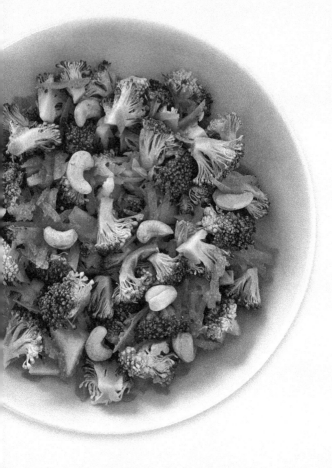

Broccoli Carrot Salad

Visual Recipe
by DAREBEE
© darebee.com

	SMALL	MEDIUM	LARGE
broccoli	1 cup ~ 150g	2 cups ~ 300g	3 cups ~ 450g
carrot	1	1	2
rice vinegar	½ tbsp	1 tbsp	1 ½ tbsp
maple syrup	½ tbsp	1 tbsp	1 ½ tbsp
mustard	½ tbsp	1 tbsp	1 ½ tbsp
water	1 tbsp	2 tbsps	3 tbsps

LEVEL UP! Add cashews.

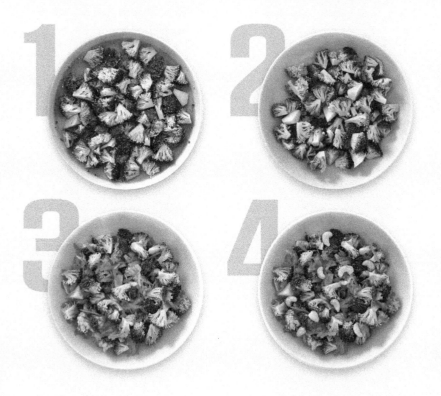

INSTRUCTIONS

1. Cut broccoli into bite-sized pieces, drizzle with vinegar and cover with plenty of water. Leave it for 10 minutes then rinse and drain.

2. Transfer rinsed and drained broccoli to a plate.

3. Add grated carrots.

4. Mix mustard, maple syrup, vinegar and water together to make the dressing. Drizzle it over the salad and mix well. Season for taste and top with cashews.

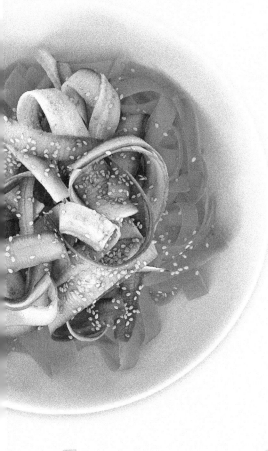

Carrot Cucumber Ribbon Salad

Visual Recipe
by DAREBEE
© darebee.com

	SMALL	MEDIUM	LARGE
carrot	1	2	3
cucumber	1	2	2
balsamic vinegar	½ tbsp	1 tbsp	1 tbsp

LEVEL UP! Add sesame seeds.

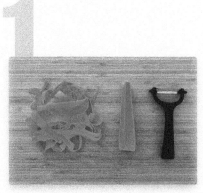
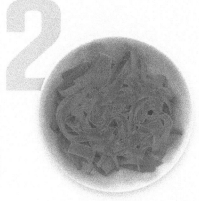
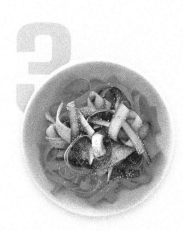

INSTRUCTIONS

1. Use a potato peeler to cut carrot and cucumber into ribbons.

2. Transfer carrots to a plate.

3. Place cucumber ribbons on top. Drizzle with vinegar, season for taste and sprinkle with sesame seeds.

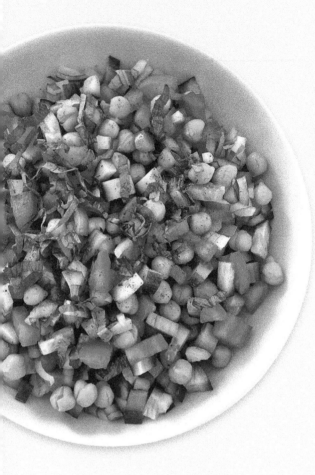

Chickpea Salad

Visual Recipe
by DAREBEE
© darebee.com

	SMALL	MEDIUM	LARGE
chickpeas	⅓ cup ~ 70g	½ cup ~ 100g	1 cup ~ 200g
tomato	1	1	2
cucumber	1	2	2
onion	1	1	1
balsamic vinegar	½ tbsp	1 tbsp	1 tbsp

LEVEL UP! Add fresh parsley and black pepper.

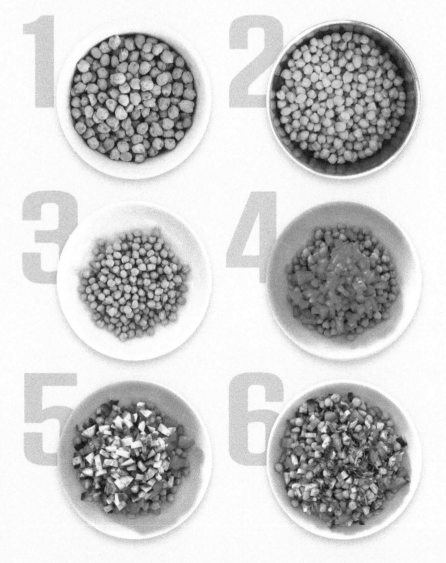

INSTRUCTIONS

1. Soak chickpeas in plenty of water overnight. The next day, rinse and drain them.

2. Place chickpeas in a cooking pot and cover with plenty of fresh water. Bring water to a boil then lower heat to low. Cover the pot with a lid and simmer chickpeas for 30 minutes. They are cooked when tender. Drain. Alternatively, use canned chickpeas: 1 can of cooked chickpeas ~ 1 cup dry.

3. Transfer drained chickpeas to a plate.

4. Add diced tomatoes.

5. Add diced cucumbers.

6. Add diced onion and drizzle with balsamic vinegar. Season for taste, mix and garnish with parsley.

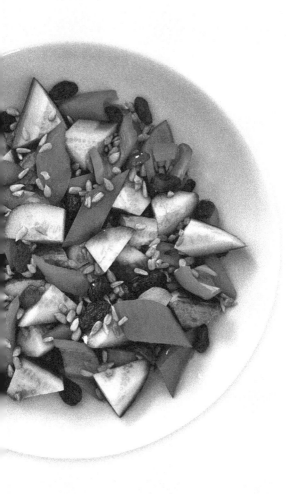

Cucumber Pepper Salad

Visual Recipe
by DAREBEE
© darebee.com

	SMALL	MEDIUM	LARGE
cucumber	1	2	3
bell peppers	1	2	3
balsamic vinegar	½ tbsp	1 tbsp	1 ½ tbsp

LEVEL UP! Add raisins, sunflower seeds and olive oil.

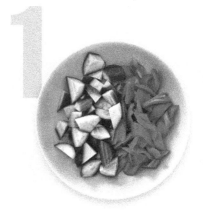
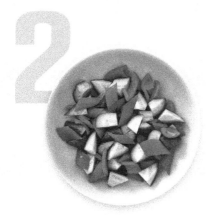
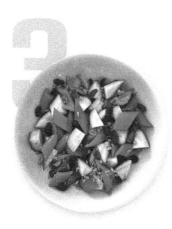

INSTRUCTIONS

1. Cut cucumbers and red bell peppers into bite-sized pieces.

2. Mix together and drizzle with balsamic vinegar and olive oil, if using. Season for taste.

3. Sprinkle with raisins and sunflower seeds.

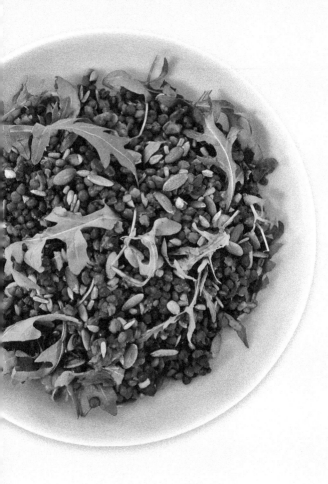

Lentil Arugula Salad

Visual Recipe by DAREBEE
© darebee.com

	SMALL	MEDIUM	LARGE
lentils	½ cup ~ 100g	1 cup ~ 200g	1 ½ cup ~ 300g
arugula	1 cup ~ 20g	1 ½ cup ~ 30g	2 cups ~ 40g
balsamic vinegar	½ tbsp	1 tbsp	1 ½ tbsp

LEVEL UP! Add sunflower and pumpkin seeds.

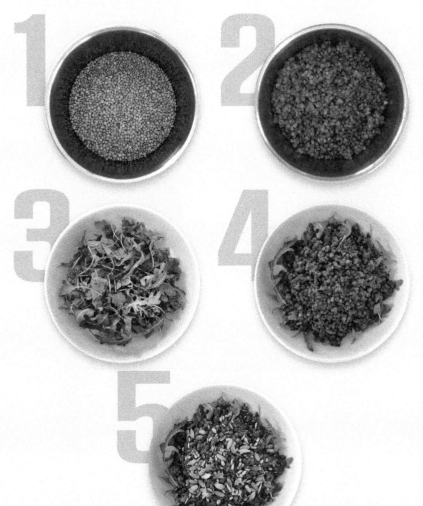

INSTRUCTIONS

1. Rinse the lentils really well.

2. Transfer the lentils to a cooking pot. Cover with double the amount of water and stir once. Bring water to a boil then lower heat to low. Cover with a lid and simmer until the lentils are tender and have completely absorbed the water ~ 30 minutes.

3. Wash and dry arugula. Add it to a plate.

4. Add cooked lentils and season for taste.

5. Drizzle with balsamic vinegar. Top with sunflower and pumpkin seeds.

SALADS

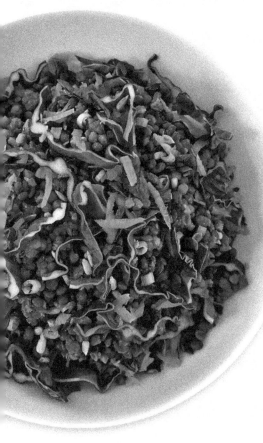

Lentil Red Cabbage Salad

Visual Recipe by DAREBEE
© darebee.com

	SMALL	MEDIUM	LARGE
lentils	½ cup ~ 100g	1 cup ~ 200g	1 ½ cup ~ 300g
red cabbage	1 cup ~ 50g	1 ½ cup ~ 75g	2 cups ~ 100g
carrot	1	1	2
balsamic vinegar	½ tbsp	1 tbsp	1 ½ tbsp

LEVEL UP! Add sunflower seeds and spring onions.

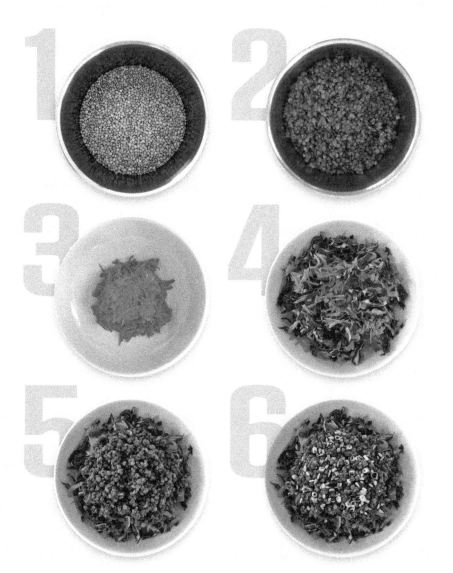

INSTRUCTIONS

1. Rinse the lentils really well.

2. Transfer the lentils to a cooking pot. Cover with double the amount of water and stir once. Bring water to a boil then lower heat to low. Cover with a lid and simmer until the lentils are tender and have completely absorbed the water ~ 30 minutes.

3. Peel and grate carrot. Add to a plate.

4. Add cut red cabbage and mix.

5. Add cooked lentils and season for taste.

6. Drizzle with balsamic vinegar and top with sunflower seeds and spring onions.

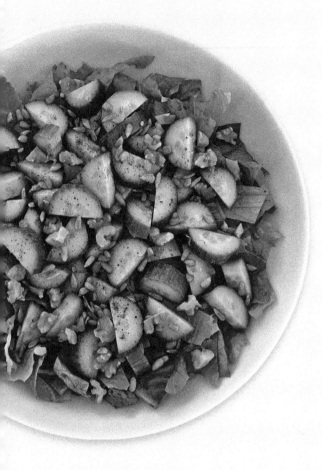

Lettuce Cucumber Salad

Visual Recipe by DAREBEE
© darebee.com

	SMALL	MEDIUM	LARGE
lettuce	2 cups ~ 100g	3 cups ~ 150g	4 cups ~ 200g
cucumber	1	2	3
olive oil	¼ tbsp	½ tbsp	1 tbsp

LEVEL UP! Add sunflower seeds and chopped walnuts.

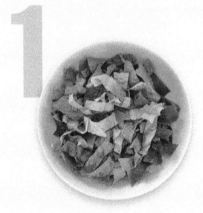 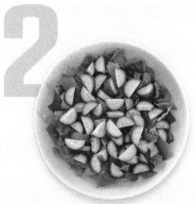 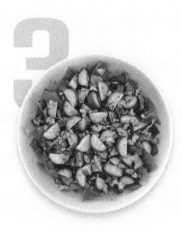

INSTRUCTIONS

1. Wash and cut lettuce. Transfer to a plate.

2. Cut cucumbers and add to the lettuce. Season for taste and mix.

3. Drizzle with olive oil and top with chopped walnuts and sunflower seeds.

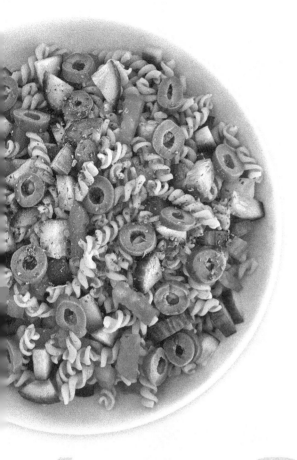

Pasta Salad

Visual Recipe
by DAREBEE
© darebee.com

	SMALL	MEDIUM	LARGE
pasta	½ cup ~ 120g	1 ½ cup ~ 180g	2 cups ~ 180g
tomato	1	1	2
cucumber	1	2	2

LEVEL UP! Add balsamic vinegar, green olives and oregano.

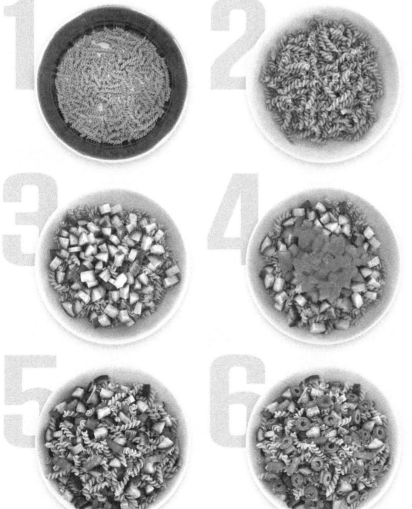

INSTRUCTIONS

1. Fill a large cooking pot with water and bring it to a boil. Add pasta and lower heat to medium. Season for taste and boil the pasta for the amount of cooking time given in its packaging instructions. Alternatively, boil it until it becomes soft and no longer crunchy.

2. Drain it and transfer to a plate.

3. Add diced cucumbers.

4. Add diced tomatoes.

5. Drizzle with balsamic vinegar and mix well.

6. Sprinkle with oregano and top with olives.

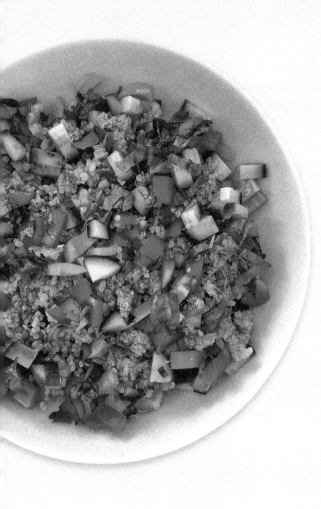

Quinoa Salad

Visual Recipe
by DAREBEE
© darebee.com

	SMALL	MEDIUM	LARGE
quinoa	⅓ cup ~ 70g	½ cup ~ 100g	1 cup ~ 200g
cucumber	1	1	1
bell peppers	2	2	2
balsamic vinegar	½ tbsp	1 tbsp	1 ½ tbsp

LEVEL UP! Add fresh parsley.

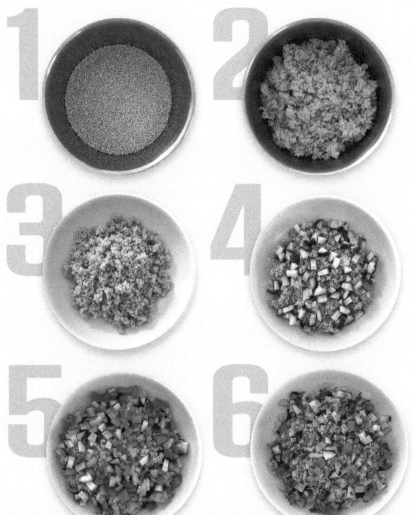

INSTRUCTIONS

1. Rinse quinoa really well.

2. Transfer the quinoa to a cooking pot. Cover with double the amount of water and stir once. Bring water to a boil then lower heat to low. Cover with a lid. Cook the quinoa until it is tender and it has completely absorbed the water ~ 15 minutes.

3. Transfer cooked quinoa to a plate.

4. Add diced cucumber.

5. Add diced bell peppers.

6. Season for taste and mix. Drizzle with balsamic vinegar and garnish with parsley.

SALADS

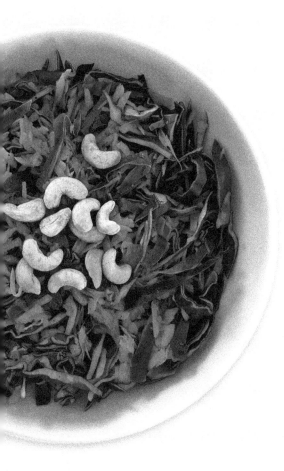

Red Cabbage Carrot Salad

Visual Recipe
by DAREBEE
© darebee.com

	SMALL	MEDIUM	LARGE
red cabbage	1 cup ~ 50g	2 cups ~ 100g	3 cups ~ 150g
carrots	1	1	2
balsamic vinegar	½ tbsp	1 tbsp	1 ½ tbsp

LEVEL UP! Add cashews.

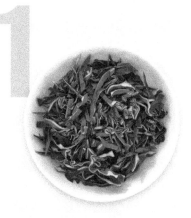
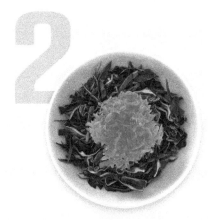
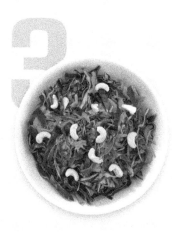

INSTRUCTIONS

1. Cut red cabbage into strips and transfer it to a plate.

2. Peel and grate carrots and add them to the cabbage.

3. Season for taste and mix. Drizzle with balsamic vinegar and top with cashews.

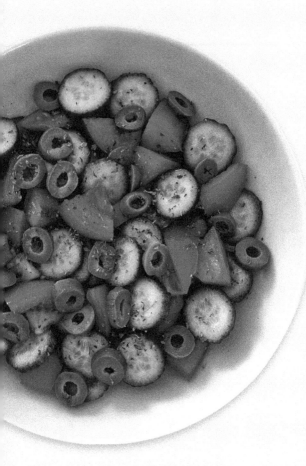

Tomato Cucumber Salad

Visual Recipe
by DAREBEE
© darebee.com

	SMALL	MEDIUM	LARGE
tomato	1	2	3
cucumber	1	2	3

LEVEL UP! Add olives, olive oil, oregano.

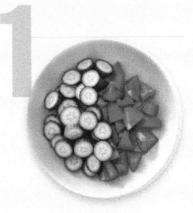

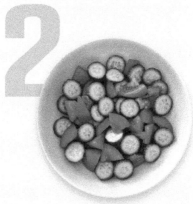

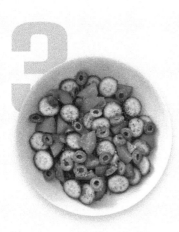

INSTRUCTIONS

1. Cut cucumbers and tomatoes into bite-sized pieces.

2. Mix together and drizzle with olive oil, if using. Season for taste.

3. Top with olives and sprinkle with oregano.

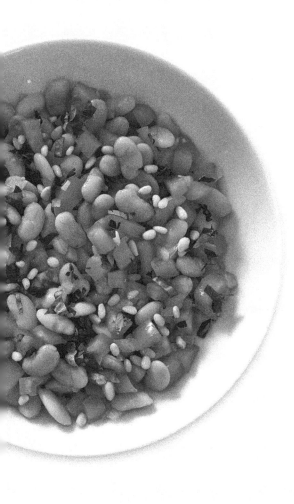

White Bean Salad

Visual Recipe
by DAREBEE
© darebee.com

	SMALL	MEDIUM	LARGE
white beans	¼ cup ~ 50g	½ cup ~ 100g	1 cup ~ 200g
tomato	1	1	2
onion	1	1	1
balsamic vinegar	1 tbsp	2 tbsps	3 tbsps
molasses	1 tsp	2 tsps	3 tsps

LEVEL UP! Add pine nuts and fresh parsley.

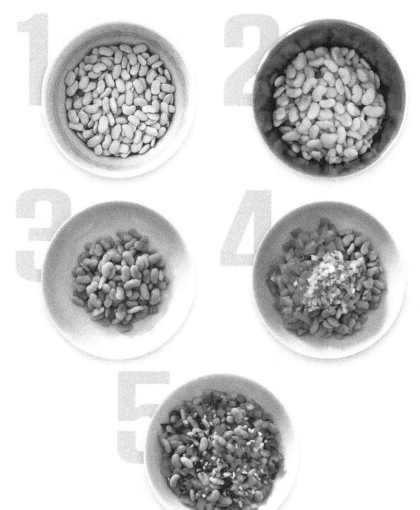

INSTRUCTIONS

1. Soak beans in plenty of water overnight. The next day, rinse and drain them. Place the beans in a cooking pot and cover with plenty of fresh water.

2. Bring water to a boil then lower heat to low. Cover the pot with a lid and set the timer for 45 minutes. They are cooked when tender. Drain the beans. Alternatively, use canned beans: 1 can of cooked beans ~ 1 cup dry.

3. Transfer drained beans to a plate.

4. Dice tomato and onion and add them to the beans.

5. Mix together balsamic vinegar with molasses and season for taste to make the dressing. Drizzle it over the beans and vegetables and mix well. Top with pine nuts and garnish with fresh parsley.

SALADS

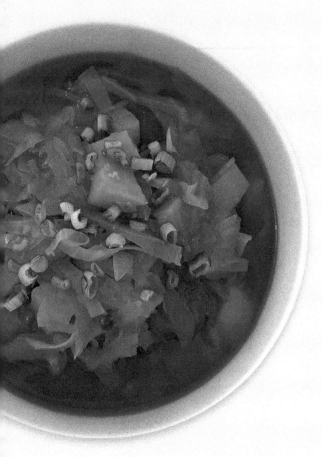

Beetroot Soup

Visual Recipe by DAREBEE
© darebee.com

	SMALL	MEDIUM	LARGE
cabbage	1 cup ~ 50g	1 ½ cup ~ 75g	2 cups ~ 100g
potato	-	1	2
beetroot	1 ~ 200g	1 ~ 200g	1 ~ 200g
onion	1	1	1
tomato paste	1 tbsp	1 tbsp	2 tbsps
water	2 cups ~ 400ml	2 ½ cups ~ 500ml	3 cups ~ 600ml

LEVEL UP! Add 2 bay leaves and spring onions.

1

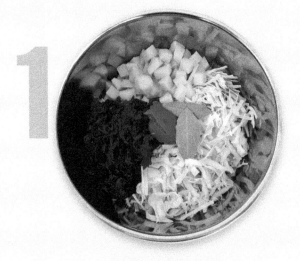

2

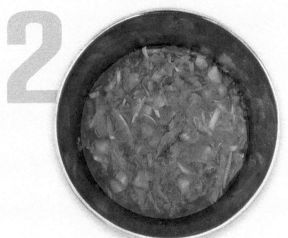

INSTRUCTIONS

1. Clean and dice the onion. Slice cabbage and grate beetroot. Add all of the ingredients to a large cooking pot, season for taste and cover with water.

2. Bring to a boil, lower the heat to low, cover the pot with a lid and simmer for 30 minutes, if using cooked beetroot; 45 minutes, if using raw beetroot. Garnish with spring onions.

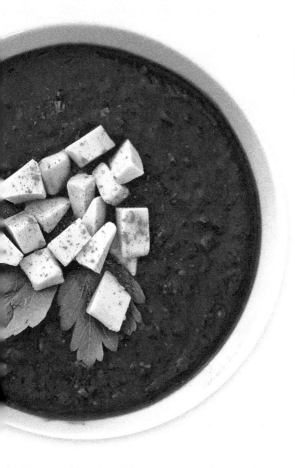

Black Bean Soup

**Visual Recipe
by DAREBEE
© darebee.com**

	SMALL	MEDIUM	LARGE
black beans	¼ cup ~ 50g	½ cup ~ 100g	1 cup ~ 200g
onion	1	1	2
tomato paste	1 tbsp	2 tbsps	3 tbsps
molasses	1 tsp	2 tsps	3 tsps
water	2 cups	3 cups	4 cups

LEVEL UP! Add avocado and fresh parsley. And add ½ tablespoon black pepper and ½ tablespoon cayenne pepper for the extra kick.

INSTRUCTIONS

1. Soak black beans in plenty of water overnight. The next day, rinse and drain them. Alternatively, use canned beans: 1 can of cooked beans ~ 1 cup dry.

2. Dice the onion. Combine all of the ingredients in a large cooking pot, season for taste and stir. Season for taste and add cayenne pepper, if using. Bring to a boil, lower the heat to low, cover the pot with a lid and let simmer for 45-60 minutes, if using soaked beans; 30 minutes, if using canned beans.

3. Use a hand blender to blend some of the soup or all of it, depending on how chunky you want it to be. Alternatively, keep it as is.

4. Garnish with diced avocado and fresh parsley.

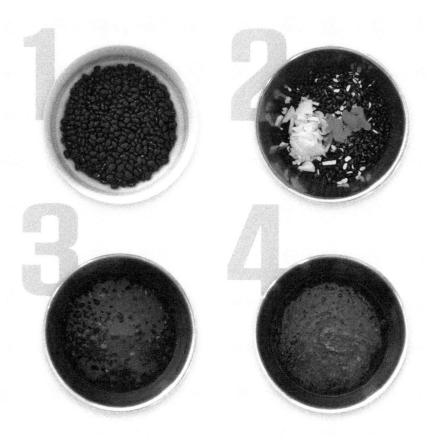

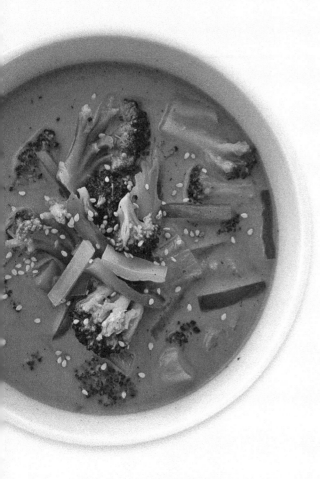

Broccoli Soup

Visual Recipe
by DAREBEE
© darebee.com

	SMALL	MEDIUM	LARGE
broccoli	1 cup ~ 150g	2 cups ~ 300g	3 cups ~ 450g
bell pepper	1	1	2
coconut milk	3oz ~ 100ml	5oz ~ 150ml	7oz ~ 200ml
tomato paste	1 tbsp	2 tbsps	3 tbsps
molasses	1 tsp	2 tsps	3 tsps
curry powder	½ tbsp	1 tbsp	1 ½ tbsp
water	1 cup ~ 200ml	2 cups ~ 400ml	2 ½ cups ~ 500ml

LEVEL UP! Add sesame seeds.

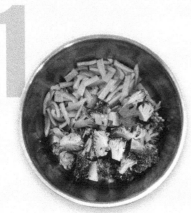
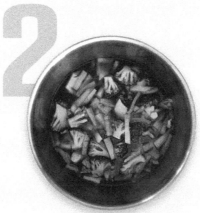
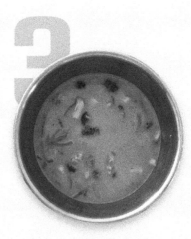

INSTRUCTIONS

1. Cut green bell pepper into strips and broccoli florets into bite-sized pieces. Combine all ingredients, except coconut milk, in a large cooking pot. Season for taste.

2. Bring to a boil, lower the heat to low. Cover the pot with a lid and let simmer for 5 minutes.

3. Add coconut milk and stir. Season for taste. Cook for another 2 minutes stirring continuously. Garnish with sesame seeds.

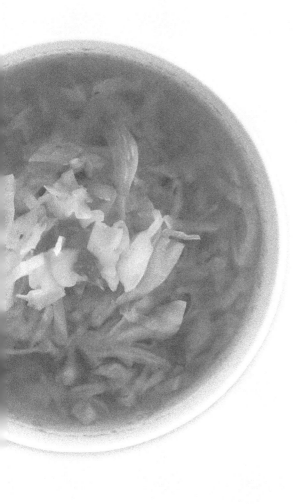

Cabbage Soup

Visual Recipe
by DAREBEE
© darebee.com

	SMALL	MEDIUM	LARGE
cabbage	1 cup ~ 50g	2 cups ~ 100g	3 cups ~ 150g
tomato	1	1	2
onion	1	1	1
water	1 cup ~ 200ml	2 cups ~ 400ml	3 cups ~ 600ml

LEVEL UP! Add garlic clove.

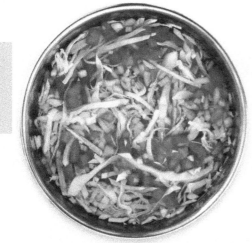

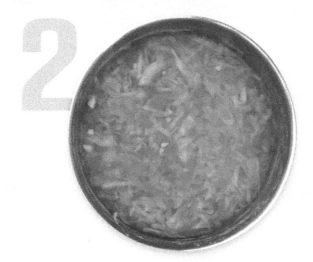

INSTRUCTIONS

1. Cut the cabbage into strips, dice the tomato, onion and garlic clove. Add all of the ingredients to a large cooking pot, season for taste and cover with water.

2. Bring to a boil, lower the heat to low, cover the pot with a lid and let simmer for 20 minutes. Serve with rice and/or bread.

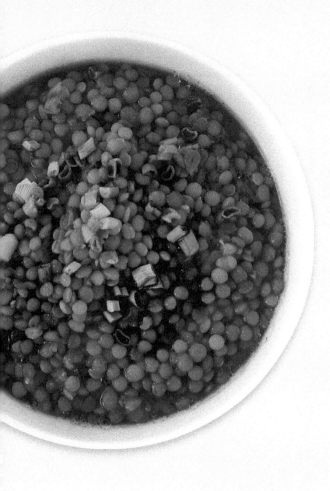

Lentil Soup

Visual Recipe
by DAREBEE
© darebee.com

	SMALL	MEDIUM	LARGE
lentils	½ cup ~ 100g	1 cup ~ 200g	1 ½ cup ~ 300g
onion	1	1	1
tomato paste	1 tbsp	1 ½ tbsp	2 tbsps
molasses	1 tsp	1 ½ tsp	2 tsps
water	2 cups ~ 400ml	3 cups ~ 600ml	4 cups ~ 800ml

LEVEL UP! Add 2 bay leaves and replace salt with soy sauce. Serve with a dash of balsamic vinegar.

1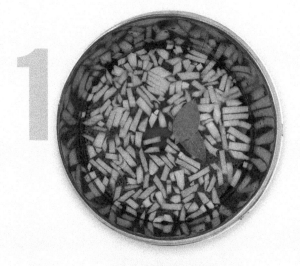

INSTRUCTIONS

1. Rinse lentils really well. Clean and dice the onion. Add all of the ingredients to a large cooking pot, season for taste and cover with water.

2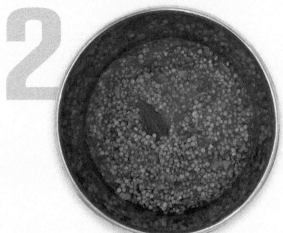

2. Bring to a boil, lower the heat to low, cover the pot with a lid and simmer for 30 minutes. The soup is ready once the lentils are tender. Garnish with spring onions.

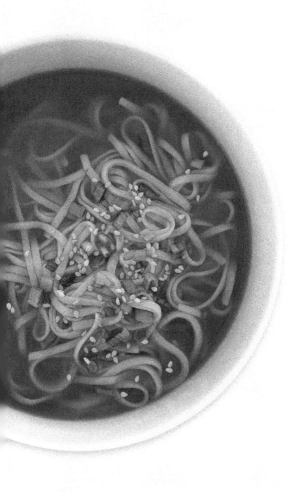

Miso Noodle Soup

Visual Recipe
by DAREBEE
© darebee.com

	SMALL	MEDIUM	LARGE
noodles	3oz ~ 80g	4oz ~ 120g	5oz ~ 160g
seaweed flakes	½ tbsp	1 tbsp	1 ½ tbsp
miso paste	½ tbsp	1 tbsp	1 ½ tbsp
water	2 cups ~ 400ml	2 ½ cups ~ 500ml	3 cups ~ 600ml

LEVEL UP! Add spring onions and sesame seeds.

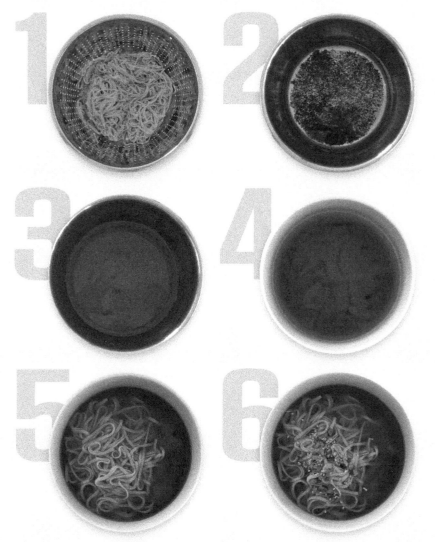

INSTRUCTIONS

1. Fill a large cooking pot with water and bring it to a boil. Add noodles and lower heat to medium. Boil the noodles for the amount of cooking time given in its packaging instructions. Usually ~ 4 minutes.

2. In a separate cooking pot bring water to a boil and add seaweed flakes to it. Reduce heat to medium and simmer for 10 minutes.

3. Remove from heat, add miso paste and whisk together until the paste completely dissolves.

4. Transfer to a bowl.

5. Add drained noodles.

6. Garnish with spring onions and sprinkle with sesame seeds.

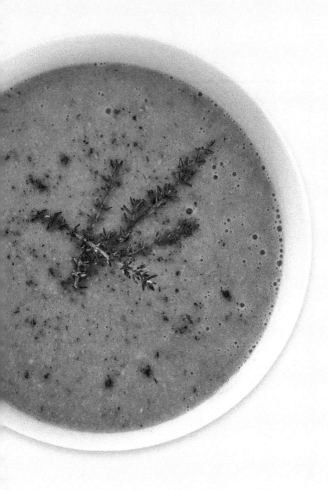

Mushroom Soup

Visual Recipe
by DAREBEE
© darebee.com

	SMALL	MEDIUM	LARGE
mushrooms	7oz ~ 200g	10oz ~ 300g	13oz ~ 400g
onion	1	1	1
milk	3oz ~ 100ml	5oz ~ 150ml	7oz ~ 200ml
flour	½ tbsp	1 tbsp	1½ tbsp
water	2 cups ~ 400ml	2½ cups ~ 500ml	3 cups ~ 600ml

LEVEL UP! Add fresh or dried thyme and black pepper.

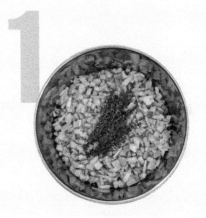
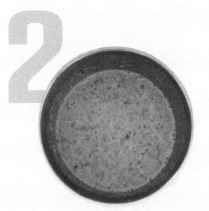
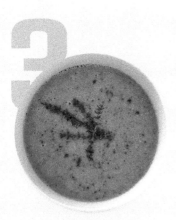

INSTRUCTIONS

1. Add diced mushrooms, onion and thyme, fresh or dry, to a pot. Add water and bring to a boil. Reduce heat, season for taste and stir. Cover with a lid and simmer for 20 minutes.

2. Mix milk with flour and add to the mushrooms. Simmer and stir for 2 minutes or until the soup thickens. Use a hand blender to blend the soup if you like it less chunky.

3. Sprinkle with black pepper and garnish with thyme.

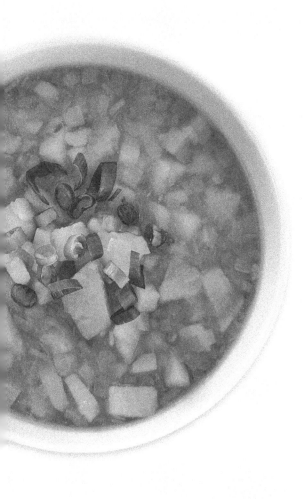

Potato & Leek Soup

Visual Recipe
by DAREBEE
© darebee.com

	SMALL	MEDIUM	LARGE
potatoes	1 medium	2 medium	3 medium
leek	1	2	2
water	2 cups ~ 400ml	2 ½ cups ~ 500ml	3 cups ~ 600ml

LEVEL UP! Add 2 bay leaves and spring onions.

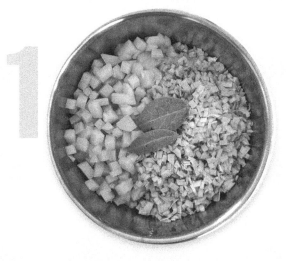

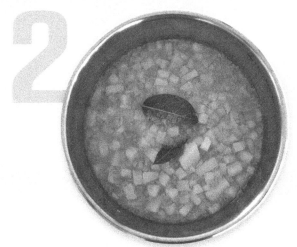

INSTRUCTIONS

1. Clean and finely dice potatoes and leek. Add both to a large cooking pot, season for taste and cover with water.

2. Bring to a boil, lower the heat to low, cover the pot with a lid and let simmer for 30 minutes. Remove bay leaves, if using. Garnish with spring onions.

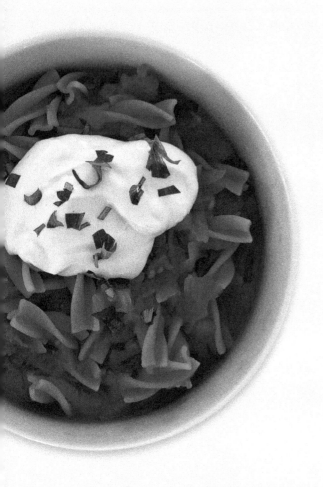

Tomato Pasta Soup

Visual Recipe
by DAREBEE
© darebee.com

	SMALL	MEDIUM	LARGE
tomato	1	2	3
onion	1	1	1
molasses	1 tsp	2 tsps	3 tsps
pasta	½ cup ~ 60g	1 cup ~ 120g	1 ½ cup ~ 180g
water	1 cup ~ 200ml	1 ½ cup ~ 300ml	2 cups ~ 400ml

LEVEL UP! Add heavy cream and fresh parsley.

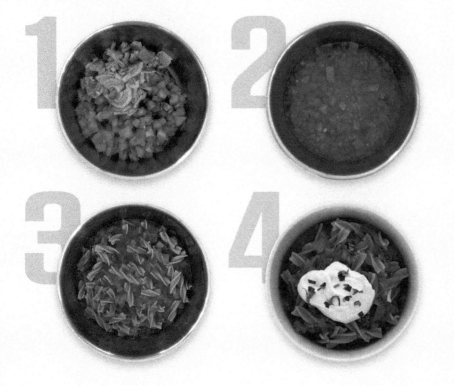

INSTRUCTIONS

1. Dice tomato and onion and add it to a large cooking pot. Add molasses and water. You can use canned chopped tomatoes instead of fresh: 1 can of chopped tomatoes ~ 2 medium tomatoes.

2. Bring to a boil, lower the heat to low, cover the pot with a lid and let simmer for 20 minutes.

3. Add pasta and stir. Season for taste. Cook for another 10 minutes or until pasta is cooked.

4. Garnish with heavy cream and fresh parsley.

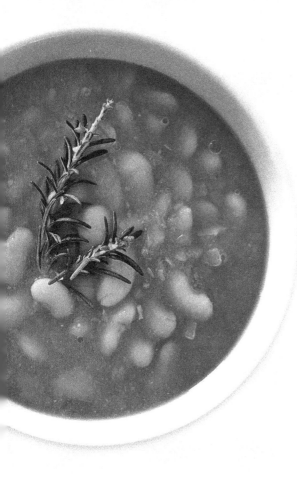

White Bean Soup

Visual Recipe
by DAREBEE
© darebee.com

	SMALL	MEDIUM	LARGE
white beans	¼ cup ~ 50g	½ cup ~ 100g	1 cup ~ 200g
carrot	1	1	2
onion	1	1	1
tomato paste	1 tbsp	2 tbsps	3 tbsps
molasses	1 tsp	2 tsps	3 tsps
water	2 cups	3 cups	4 cups

LEVEL UP! Add fresh or dried rosemary.

INSTRUCTIONS

1. Soak beans in plenty of water overnight. The next day, rinse and drain them. Alternatively, use canned beans: 1 can of cooked beans ~ 1 cup dry.

2. Finely dice onion and carrots. Combine all of the ingredients in a large cooking pot, season for taste and stir. Add fresh or dried rosemary, if using. Bring to a boil, lower the heat to low, cover the pot with a lid and let simmer for: 30 minutes, if using canned beans; 45 minutes, if using soaked beans.

3. Use a hand blender to blend some of the soup or all of it, depending on how chunky you want it to be. Alternatively, keep it as is.

4. Garnish with fresh rosemary.

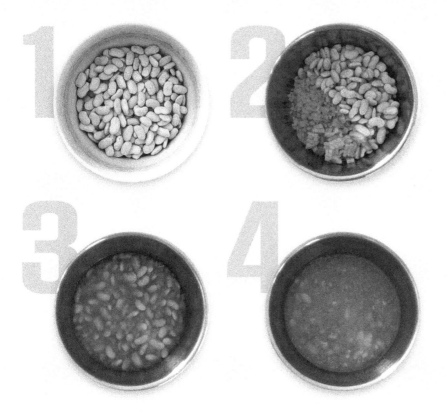

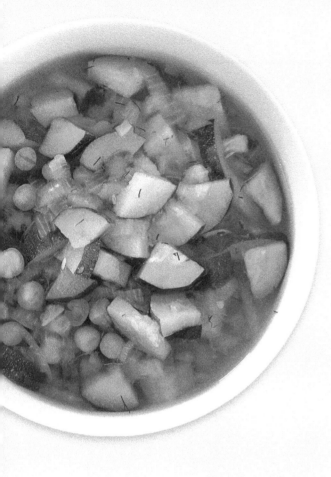

Zucchini Soup

Visual Recipe
by DAREBEE
© darebee.com

	SMALL	MEDIUM	LARGE
zucchini	1	2	2
peas	½ cup ~ 80g	1 cup ~ 160g	1 ½ cup ~ 240g
onion	1	1	1
carrot	1	1	1
water	1 cup ~ 200ml	1 ½ cup ~ 300ml	2 cups ~ 400ml

LEVEL UP! Add dried dill.

1

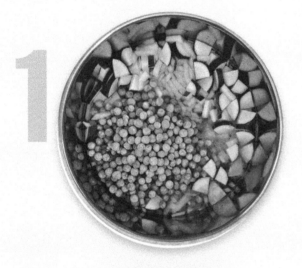

INSTRUCTIONS

1. Dice zucchini and onions, peel and grate carrot. Add all of the ingredients to a large cooking pot, season for taste and cover with water.

2

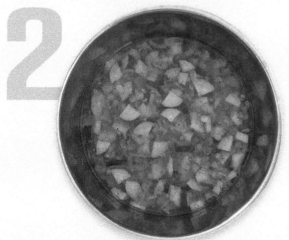

2. Bring to a boil, lower the heat to low, cover the pot with a lid and let simmer for 30 minutes. Serve with rice and/or bread.

A (Very) Brief Guide To The Science of Taste

The sensors in our mouths that detect basic tastes such as sweet, salty, bitter, sour and umami, and arguably a few others are only the start of the story on how the body detects and processes the sensory signal we call "taste".

The way the brain represents these tastes is just as important. Researchers have recently developed a 'gustotopic map' based on the idea that, just as each taste bud on the tongue responds to a single taste, so there are regions of the brain that are similarly dedicated to the recognition and processing of these signals.

The other recent revelation in taste research is that the receptors that detect bitter, sweet and umami are not restricted to the tongue. They are distributed throughout the stomach, intestine and pancreas, where they aid the digestive process by influencing appetite and regulating insulin production. They have also been found in the airways, where they have an impact on respiration, and even on sperm, where they affect maturation.

Researchers are working on acquiring a better understanding of what they do and how they work which will have implications, in future,for treating conditions ranging from diabetes to infertility.

Because the brain is a massively networked associative data machine designed to make sense of everything it senses; taste has been found to also play a role in memory, emotion and learning. Unsurprisingly, what science is discovering about our sense of taste is intricately linked with our sense of physical identity, our knowledge of the world and our understanding of how we fit in it.

Fitness is a journey, not a destination.
- Darebee Project

Thank you!

Thank you for purchasing Hey, I Can Make It! - Plant-Based DAREBEE Cook Book. DAREBEE is a non-profit global fitness resource dedicated to making fitness and health, in all their different formats, accessible for everyone, no matter their circumstances. The project is supported exclusively via user donations and book royalties.

After printing costs and store fees every book developed by the DAREBEE project makes approximately $1 and it goes directly into our project maintenance and development fund.

Each sale helps us keep the DAREBEE resource growing, maintain it and keep it up. Thank you for making a difference in its future!

Other DAREBEE books

100 No-Equipment Workouts Vol 1.

100 No-Equipment Workouts Vol 2.

100 No-Equipment Workouts Vol 3.

100 Office Workouts: No Equipment, No-Sweat, Fitness Mini-Routines
You Can Do At Work.

Pocket Workouts: 100 no-equipment workouts

ABS 100 Workouts: Visual Easy-To-Follow ABS Exercise Routines
for All Fitness Levels

100 HIIT Workouts: Visual easy-to-follow routines for all fitness levels

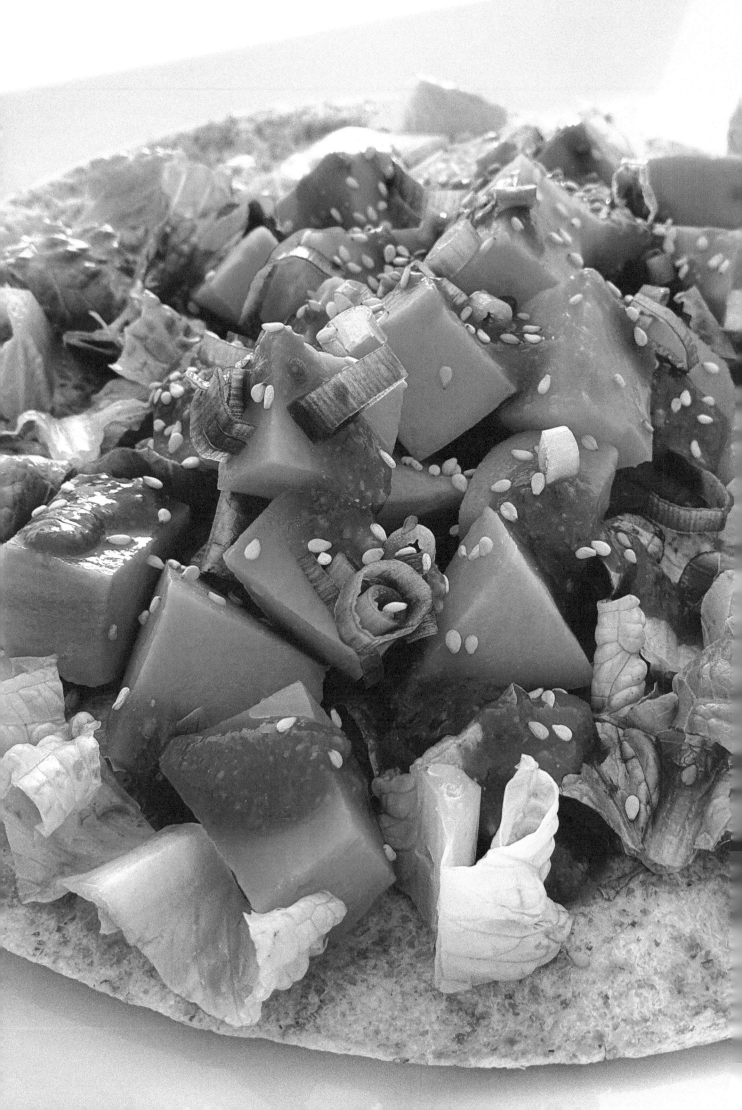

Notes & Shortcuts For Your Favorite Recipes

Notes & Shortcuts For Your Favorite Recipes

Notes & Shortcuts For Your Favorite Recipes

Notes & Shortcuts For Your Favorite Recipes

Notes & Shortcuts For Your Favorite Recipes

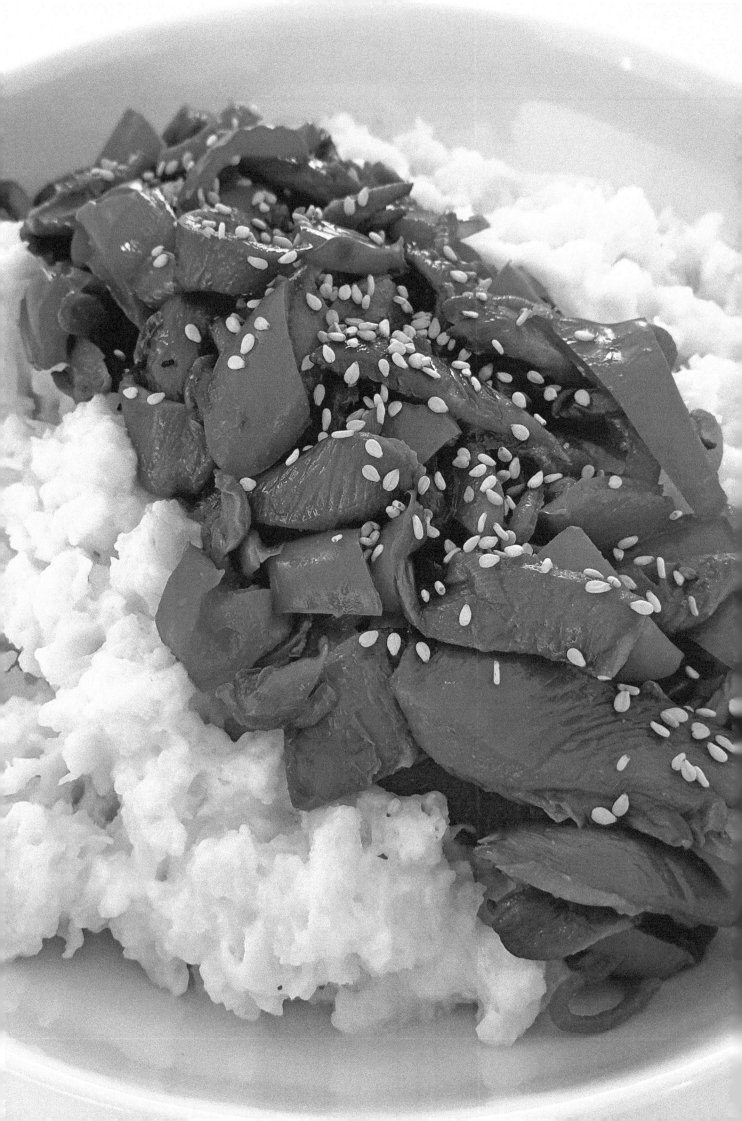

Lightning Source UK Ltd.
Milton Keynes UK
UKHW050308160121
377025UK00008B/43